W9-BQC-659

LIVING WITH JUVENILE ARTHRITIS

A Parent's Guide

Kimberly Poston Miller

SpryPublishing
ideas to life

American Fork Library

Copyright © 2013 Kimberly Poston Miller

All rights reserved under International and
Pan American Copyright Conventions.

No part of this book may be reproduced or transmitted in any form or by
any means electronic or mechanical including photocopying, recording, or by
any information storage and retrieval system, without permission in writing
from the publisher.

This edition is published by Spry Publishing LLC
2500 South State Street
Ann Arbor, MI 48104 USA

Printed and bound in the United States of America.

10   9   8   7   6   5   4   3   2   1

Library of Congress Control Number: 2013937936

Paperback ISBN: 978-1-938170-24-9
eBook ISBN: 978-1-938170-25-6

Disclaimer: Spry Publishing LLC does not assume responsibility for the contents
or opinions expressed herein. Although every precaution is taken to ensure that
information is accurate as of the date of publication, differences of opinion exist.
The opinions expressed herein are those of the author and do not necessarily
reflect the views of the publisher. The information contained in this book is not
intended to replace professional advisement of an individual's doctor prior to
beginning or changing an individual's course of treatment.

This book is dedicated to my sons,
along with the hundreds of thousands of children
who bravely battle this disease every day—
you are my heroes.

Contents

Foreword   6
Introduction   9

Part 1 Learning the Ropes
Chapter 1   A Decade of Diagnosis   15
Chapter 2   The Game Changer   31
Chapter 3   An Unpredictable Opponent   44
Chapter 4   The Team Approach   63
Chapter 5   The Head Coach   88
Chapter 6   Controlling JA   102
                   and Handling Flares
Chapter 7   Pain Management   115

Part 2 Life Goes On
Chapter 8   Family Matters   129
Chapter 9   Your Cheering Section   144
Chapter 10   Back to School   168
Chapter 11   The Whole Child   185
Chapter 12   Too Many Hats   207
Chapter 13   Playing It Day by Day   228
Chapter 14   Getting Involved   237

Resources   252
Appendix   259
Acknowledgments   261
Index   263

Foreword

These days, whenever I turn on the TV or pick up a newspaper, there's a story about "autoimmunity" or "autoimmune disease." But that was not always the case. When I founded the American Autoimmune Related Diseases Association, Inc. (AARDA) back in 1990, these terms were not part of the public dialogue.

Juvenile arthritis (JA) is one of the many autoimmune conditions that are increasing at a rapid rate. Often misunderstood as an "older person's" affliction, or just aches and pains, the general public doesn't always understand that this disease is an autoimmune condition that can affect children from infants to teens.

Whether juvenile arthritis, multiple sclerosis, celiac disease, psoriasis, type 1 diabetes, or Graves' disease, the pathology is the same—a malfunctioning immune system. When you're healthy, your immune system creates an army of antibodies that fight off foreign invaders such as viruses and bacteria. When you have an autoimmune disease (AD), your immune system creates the same kind of army, only it mistakenly recognizes healthy tissue and organs as foreign invaders and attacks them, producing disease.

Autoimmune diseases, whether rheumatic, dermatologic, or endocrine, share a genetic background so they tend to run in families. They also cluster in individual patients. Thus, it is not uncommon for patients to have multiple ADs. Of the more than 50 million Americans who live and cope with these diseases, many of them are children. Today, roughly 100

ADs have been identified. Together, they are responsible for more than $100 billion in direct healthcare costs annually.

I've heard it said AD is not common in children. Our experience at AARDA has been quite the opposite. Over the years, we've heard from many parents with children who have been diagnosed with ADs. The problem is there haven't been many epidemiological studies on ADs in children (or adults, for that matter), so there is no accurate tracking of the numbers of kids actually affected. Like adults with ADs, getting a proper diagnosis for a child with an AD can be a frustrating and lengthy process that takes years with many visits to various specialists.

Parents of children with ADs also face a unique set of challenges and frustrations. I would say the biggest challenge is overseeing and coordinating their care because, ultimately, this responsibility lies with the parents. Children, like adults, often have multiple ADs. For example, a child with lupus (a condition under the juvenile arthritis umbrella) may also have type 1 diabetes. The rheumatologist treating the lupus may want to put the child on steroids, which is not as desirable to the endocrinologist treating the diabetes, since steroids can affect blood sugar levels. It is then up to the parents to make the decision and resolve this treatment conflict. And it's not an easy choice.

Making decisions about the new therapies available to treat ADs such as JA is also a challenge. Many of these therapies have not yet been tested in children. They may have a high benefit, but they also come with some degree of risk. Again, something parents must weigh and then decide.

Frustration is also part of the equation. I've talked to parents whose children have Crohn's disease, for example, who are at their wit's end because the child's teachers don't seem to realize the urgency and potential embarrassment involved with this disease. When a child raises his or her hand and says they need to use the bathroom, they mean they need to use the bathroom *now*. If this happens repeatedly throughout the day, and if the teacher remarks on it, the class can become involved and the ridicule can start. It's a very unfortunate situation.

I raise my glass to the parents who find themselves raising a child with juvenile arthritis or any other autoimmune disease. It is a difficult task, there are no clear cut directions to follow, and no one "right" way to proceed. It can be overwhelming, at best.

Living with Juvenile Arthritis: A Parent's Guide helps families find their way through this uncharted territory, with solid advice from families who have been there. From actual disease management to ancillary lifestyle changes and situational advice unique to childhood, Kimberly Poston Miller's book will not disappoint parents who are looking for guidance on managing more than the medical portion of their child's disease; it is a guide to healing the whole child and learning to live, and even thrive, under these difficult circumstances.

Virginia T. Ladd
Founder and President
American Autoimmune Related Diseases Association

Introduction

So your child has been diagnosed with juvenile arthritis. Now what? I know you may be feeling sad, angry, confused, and helpless. I remember those feelings well. I also remember wishing for a step-by-step instruction manual. Unfortunately, like most things in life, this diagnosis doesn't come with directions. If you're looking for a medical guide, you've come to the wrong place. However, if you're looking for answers to some of the other tough questions faced by parents of children with juvenile arthritis (JA), I can help you find them.

I can help you because I'm one of you. I have two children diagnosed with different forms of JA, and although I'm not a doctor or nurse, I often joke about being a medical paraprofessional. Just ask my pediatrician! And, I guarantee that over the coming weeks, months, or even years, you'll find yourself becoming one as well. Let me also assure you that you'll do better than you think you can.

Although every case of JA is different, many of the issues are the same. I learned so much "the hard way," which is why I decided to write this book. By sharing my family's experiences with you, I hope I can help you avoid a few common mistakes, provide some much-needed support, and help you make peace with this diagnosis—in *all* aspects of your child's life. My wish is that this book will guide you through those unknown and sometimes frightening days after diagnosis, as well as the long and twisty road ahead. I want to help you learn to deal with the medical community effectively, so you can build a good healthcare team and make sense of insurance issues. I want to give you the tools you need to soften the impact your child's condition will have on family and friends and help you deal with the emotional roller coaster you will inevitably face. I want to teach you to create good social and educational opportunities for your children if circumstances become difficult. Most importantly, I want to help you lessen the toll this disease can have on your children—both the ones who are ill, and the ones who are not—because this diagnosis is a family affair.

As parents, we have many roles: teacher, chauffeur, chef, playmate, disciplinarian, and, of course, medical caregiver. Even with a child who has no chronic illness, you have been filling this important position and are more experienced than you think! Before any diagnosis, you were administering routine medical care. You've already performed basic first aid on bumps and scrapes, determined when a fever was too high, or when that cough was hanging on just a little too long. You've been the one to decide when it's time to see the doctor or get outside care. When you have a child with a chronic illness, this role does not change, it just magnifies significantly.

Depending on the severity of your child's case, you may find yourself administering injections or keeping track of multiple medications, sometimes feeling as though you have earned the credentials of an NCNA (**Non**-*certified* nurse's aide). You will become the first to recognize subtle changes in your child's health or condition and relay the "right" information to your child's medical team. You are going to be the first point of care even with skilled doctors in your corner. In other words, you'll be the bridge between your child and his or her medical care.

After the shock of the initial diagnosis wears off and you become more comfortable with the medical aspects, you'll find that's just the beginning. The other challenges you face as a parent become magnified as well—from balancing the needs of your marriage and other children, to special educational considerations, and adjustments to your day-to-day life. You will also take on some new roles, including makeshift social worker, surrogate pal, and head cheerleader for your child. It can be overwhelming.

A Game Plan

As a former National Football League (NFL) wife and mother of two athletic sons (yes, even with JA!), I have learned a lot from sports. As you can imagine, sports are *huge* in our home. We watch them, we play them, and they have shaped our frame of reference. Thanks to sports, I know the value of a good team, a great game plan, and an experienced coach. I have learned never to give up, despite the odds, and to adjust to ever-changing opponents. This lifestyle and these lessons have helped my family cope with the chronic illnesses faced by my children. I don't claim to know all the rules (because they seem to change constantly), but I have learned a great deal over the last ten years that I hope to share with you.

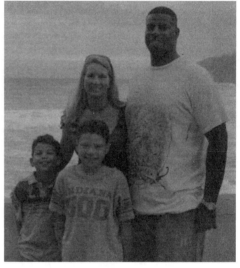

The three most important things to remember are (1) you are not alone, (2) you can do this, and (3) you will be stronger for it. Now let me help you plan your strategy for this new "season" in your child's life!

PART ONE

Learning the Ropes

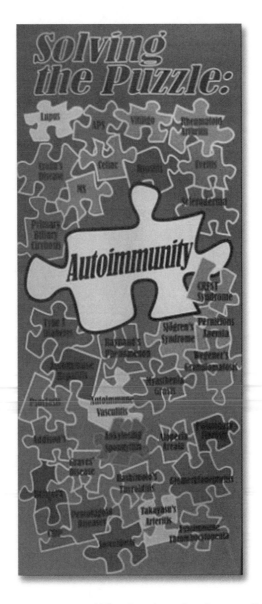

This poster conveys a message of The American Autoimmune Related Diseases Association (AARDA), the only national nonprofit health agency dedicated to bringing a national focus to autoimmunity, the major cause of serious chronic diseases. Photo courtesy of Sharon L. Harris, AARDA.

CHAPTER ONE

A Decade of Diagnosis

Pieces of the Puzzle

Anyone who has worked on a puzzle knows the satisfying feeling you get when those last few pieces fall into place. Until then, the image is often unrecognizable. Individually, the pieces may look generic and meaningless, but each one is necessary to form the complete picture. Diagnosing juvenile arthritis is a lot like that process.

If your child has been diagnosed with any form of juvenile arthritis (JA), you know it isn't always a straightforward process. JA is often difficult to diagnose and can take weeks, months, or even years to determine definitively. Unlike many other medical conditions, there is no single test and no series of lab tests that will prove or disprove the presence of juvenile arthritis. In addition, JA is a sneaky opponent—sometimes it will show itself, and sometimes it won't. To complicate matters further, there are many different forms of JA, all with diverse manifestations. Symptoms can be obvious or subtle, reactive or always present. JA has no steadfast rules, no absolute checklists, and no giant arrow that points to your child and says, "*This* kid has arthritis!" Every child is unique and, therefore, so is the path from onset to diagnosis and treatment.

To determine if a child has any form of JA, his or her healthcare provider must rely on information provided from a number of resources. Lab tests can be useful—blood work can prove the existence of some issues, but often a rheumatologic condition can be present *without* abnormal labs. Genetic testing is also helpful, but it does not determine the presence or the absence of a condition. It merely indicates the increased or decreased likelihood that a child may develop the illness. Familial history, parental input, and observation of the child all play a role in determining whether or not a child is suffering from juvenile arthritis. Discovery usually comes from repeated physical exams, a thorough medical history, and evaluation by a pediatric rheumatologist. All the pieces of the puzzle must be collected and then assembled by a healthcare practitioner before a definitive diagnosis can be made. For some, this can happen in a matter of days. For others, like our family, it can take months or even years.

COMMON SYMPTOMS OF JA

Children with juvenile arthritis may exhibit a variety of symptoms with various degrees of severity, which can make diagnosis difficult. Though not every child will experience these warning signs, the most common symptoms of JA include:

- swollen, tender and/or warm joints
- stiffness, especially in the morning or after periods of rest
- fevers
- rashes
- fatigue
- inflammation of the eye(s)
- slow or decreased growth
- joint contractures (shortening of a muscle that causes decreased joint movement or range of motion)
- pain

Grant's Diagnosis–A Tale of Ten Years

Clues from a Toddler

To say things were crazy would be an understatement. In the fall of 2000, when my son Grant was turning two, our family was coping with several major changes, including the birth of our second child, a cross-country move, and a new employer for my husband, Fred, who had just joined the Tennessee Titans. We were renting and looking for a "permanent" home, becoming acquainted with an unfamiliar area, making new friends, and, of course, adjusting to the latest addition to our family. It seemed as though we were always on the go and enjoying very little downtime. Changing teams also meant a heavier media schedule with lots of extra appearances for both Fred on his own and us as a couple. There was never a dull moment.

Grant had always been a "go-with-the-flow" kind of baby. As an NFL kid, he was accustomed to crazy schedules and a good deal of travel, along with strange people and places. However, the most recent changes really threw him for a loop. At least, that's what I thought it was at the time.

My sweet, bubbly baby boy was growing up. Barely out of diapers, he had a mind of his own and would tell me exactly what was on it. A few days after coming home from the hospital with his brother, he informed me that I was Evan's mommy now, and he "had no more mommy." He also missed his Dad, who was around more frequently during the off-season. NFL players often work 80 plus hours a week during the football season, and Grant was just too young to understand why his father was home so much, and then just wasn't. Fred being on a new team took time from me as well, as the new guy and his wife are usually desirable guests on the charity and fund-raising circuits as ambassadors for the team. Even though I was still a stay-at-home mom, a new baby and added commitments were dividing my attention—things had drastically changed for my little guy.

So, I was not entirely surprised when Grant started to become crabby and acting out more often. Our pediatrician was new to us since the relocation, and his response to Grant's huge shift in attitude was "welcome to the terrible twos" and a suggestion that we give him time to adjust. Considering all the big changes we had just made, coupled with the onset of the toddler era, I thought the doc was probably right, and things would get back to normal. I was confident that his irritability would work itself out with time, love, and patience. But, it didn't.

It felt as though I brought someone else's child with us when we moved from St. Louis. Previously an excellent traveler, Grant would no longer tolerate his car seat, often arching his back or sobbing the entire time he was strapped in. I would grit my teeth and bear it, thinking it was just a stage. Besides, I had to do what was right and keep him safe. But it wasn't just the car seat. I began to notice other things. He would squirm and complain about his high chair, and riding in the double stroller was a no-go. He would lie down to watch television. In fact, he would rather lie down than sit—*anytime, anywhere.* That's when the first warning bell went off in my mind.

As I began to watch him closer, I noticed that sometimes he would hobble like a little old man, with his hand on his lower back, slightly stooped over. And yet at other times, he walked and played just like he always had. Although I tried to talk to him about this behavior, it's difficult for a toddler to accurately explain what he or she is experiencing. Most of the time, Grant would simply say his back hurt or he had "owies," but then act completely fine. While my concern blossomed, the pain didn't seem consistent enough to be "real," except when he was doing something he didn't want to do (like being confined in the stroller, car seat, or high chair). I vacillated among thinking it was a ploy for more attention, typical terrible-twos behavior, or something that was seriously wrong. It was time to approach the pediatrician again.

This time, the doctor didn't attribute Grant's behavioral changes to the terrible twos. He suggested that in his very normal attempts to shift attention off his baby brother and back onto himself, he might simply be imitating his father's behavior. Well, kind of. While my husband obviously didn't cry every time he put on his seat belt, he *did* lie down on the couch to watch TV, exhausted at the end of the day from the physicality of his work. Every Monday (or Tuesday if there was a Monday night game) he *would* hobble around the house, battered and bruised from the game he had played the day before, often limping or holding his lower back.

Other possible explanations for Grant's strange gait and discomfort included growing pains and soreness from playing or roughhousing, especially after playdates with other rowdy teammates' kids. Intellectually, I wanted to believe these innocent explanations. It made sense—toddlers *do* imitate their parents. He *did* play hard. He *was* growing. And, since Evan was only a few months old, he *did* take up much of my time. Grant had been through a lot of big changes, and it would be normal for him to try to get my attention any way he could. It was all very logical but, in my heart, I think I knew it was more.

How Could This Happen?

When the off-season rolled around and Fred wasn't doing the "grandpa shuffle" around the house every week, Grant's behavior didn't change. My husband and I were in the middle of launching a new foundation in Middle Tennessee to help at-risk mothers and newborns when I offhandedly mentioned Grant's behavior to a colleague. She was a pediatrician who had agreed to become our pro bono medical director. Her response shocked me. While she remained calm and quiet, her demeanor indicated this was serious. She felt our son should be evaluated at Vanderbilt Children's Hospital very soon, because the type of changes and symptoms I described were *not* acceptable or common for a two year old, even under the circumstances.

The next few weeks were a blur. I was numb, terrified that I could have overlooked something that could potentially affect my child's ability to survive. I hated myself when they told me he needed an MRI of his spine to rule out a tumor and blood work to make sure it wasn't cancer. How could this happen? How did I allow it? How long did I let it go while it was taking hold of my baby?

As they say, hindsight is 20/20. At the time, I thought I did all the right things. I took him to the doctor and justified the explanations. They were all very plausible. No one wants to believe their child is "the one."

When you have a healthy baby, with no other problems, you never think the bad stuff you read about can happen to you, but it can.

As I was battling my guilt over not knowing sooner, and not taking action when I heard that first nagging voice in the back of my head, we got some good news. The lab tests ruled out cancer, and the MRI showed no abnormal mass or tumor. They did notice a few abnormalities in Grant's spine, but recommended we see an orthopedist, who then referred us to a rheumatologist. We learned that some of Grant's vertebrae were compressed, and his muscles were thickened and shortened on either side of his spine. The labs they did for rheumatologic conditions were normal, but his MRI findings, physical exam, and symptoms still worried the rheumatologist.

We were referred to a physical therapist, and Grant was started on a regimen of nonsteroidal anti-inflammatory drugs (NSAIDs). We held this course for almost a year. When all of his symptoms vanished, the rheumatologist told us to keep an eye on him, and if his symptoms came back we should be seen again. She didn't feel he had a true case of autoimmune disease; so monitoring him at home was the best option. There was a good chance that, with his normal lab work and "new" alignment, all the original problems were mechanical in nature and may not ever bother him again. We were released from the practice, happy and confident that Grant's issues were behind us.

Out of Sight, Out of Mind

We had almost seven years of smooth sailing. Well, seven years on the rheumatology front, that is. We had many years of normal childhood with all the regular ups and downs one would expect. Grant was thriving. He was doing well in school, playing team sports, and generally happy. At nine, he was a fairly big kid for his age, which came as no surprise with an offensive lineman for a dad! In general, things had been going very well. We hadn't given a second thought to his possible diagnosis, but then slowly things began to change.

In the fourth grade, Grant started to complain of ankle pain. He was shooting up like a weed, so we assumed it was just growing pains. However, the stiffness and pain were getting worse, affecting his ability to walk to school in the mornings, especially if he had played sports the day before. Since Grant was never really a complainer, I took his concerns seriously, but didn't want to overreact. I addressed the issue with his new pediatrician (we had since moved to the Chicago area) and took the steps they suggested to alleviate his pain.

By the time he started fifth grade, his ankles weren't any better despite visits to the doctor, podiatrist, and orthopedist. The general consensus was that the problem was mechanical in nature, but I had my doubts. Custom orthotics weren't making a difference, and he was starting to have back pain as well. I also noticed that Grant wasn't doing as well in school, and the boys he previously towered over were catching up or overtaking him in height. Since he was prepubescent, I didn't think too much about the sluggish growth at the time. He was so close to puberty, and slow growth before the big spurt is pretty common. Besides, everyone matures at a different rate in the tween years. Yet, given his history and the fact that other treatments were not making positive changes, our pediatrician agreed it was time to see a rheumatologist again, just in case.

Seeing a pediatric rheumatologist is not easy. We were stunned to find that the wait to be seen, even with a referral, can be months due to a shortage of practitioners in the field. Grant did get lucky and was able to see a pediatric rheumatologist on a cancellation, about two months after our initial inquiry, just as he was starting the sixth grade. We secured the earlier visit with the help of our pediatrician, who was insistent on his being seen. In many practices, the wait for a new patient can often be in excess of six to nine months!

Living in Chicago, we were lucky to have an excellent team of rheumatologists in our own backyard. Grant had more testing done, and his rheumatology labs were still in the normal ranges. Because he was an athlete playing multiple sports, we couldn't rule out mechanical issues, stress injuries, or just plain growing pains. However, given his history, rheumatology did want to follow him and help us manage the pain. Grant started on another course of NSAIDs, physical therapy, and rest from sports.

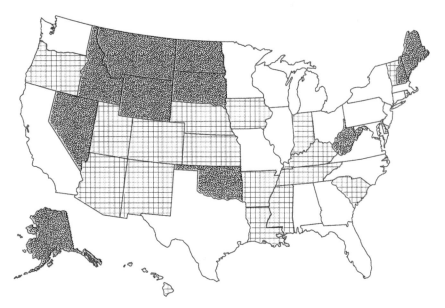

Arthritis is a disabling and painful disease that affects 50 million Americans, including 300,000 children. Nearly 1 in 250 children are living with a form of arthritis. Currently, there are less than 250 board-certified practicing pediatric rheumatologists in the United States and about 90 percent of those are clustered in and around large cities. As illustrated on the map, there are currently 11 states (dotted) that do not have a single board-certified practicing pediatric rheumatologist, 19 states (lines) with three or less, and the remaining states have 4 or more. Source information from the Arthritis Foundation.

From Bad to Worse

Despite our combined efforts to alleviate his suffering with the mildest drugs and therapy, things just continued to get worse. As the weather got colder, the pain escalated. His back hurt so badly that he would wake up in the middle of the night in excruciating pain, unable to get out of bed unassisted. Since my husband was a pro athlete, frequently dealing with chronic pain/injuries, we had the ability to give alternating hot tub/ice bath soaks in our own home. It was helpful, but definitely no fun. By the time the holidays rolled around, Grant was rarely sleeping more than an hour or two at a time, and he was begging for ice baths in the middle of the night, just to take the edge off the pain. I *knew* this was more than mechanics or sports. Seeing your child in that much pain regularly is almost beyond the scope of what any parent can take. We needed to find out what was going on and fast.

As Grant worked his way up to unbearable pain levels, rheumatology had changed his medications several times, in the hopes that a different drug would be more effective. Most of these medications take a few days or weeks to kick in, so we would hold our breath, watch, wait, and hope for *any* relief. It didn't come. After a round of the flu made its way through our house, things seemed to accelerate in the wrong direction. Even though the virus was gone, Grant never felt that much better. He was in even worse pain than before, his back would stay red and hot, and he was running low-grade fevers of "nonspecific origin."

I was advised to take him to the emergency room (ER) at the children's hospital when I thought he was at the height of his pain, in the hopes that labs taken during an episode would give the doctors better insight into the root of his condition. The ER doctors observed all the same things I did at home—swollen and red ankles, extreme sensitivity and excess warmth near his spine, but *no* abnormal lab results. He was a mystery.

To tell you the truth, at this point I didn't even care about a diagnosis. The only thing that mattered was finding a way to relieve Grant's pain. Watching your child suffer, with no end in sight and no treatments that seem to work, is something I wouldn't wish on my worst enemy. The days dragged on like years. We were sleep deprived and emotionally spent, completely wrapped up in Grant; finding him relief and finding a way for him to get better. I think these may have been our darkest days.

The Problem Revealed

At this point, the possibility of juvenile arthritis, specifically spondyloarthropathy and juvenile idiopathic arthritis (JIA), was mentioned, but my focus was less on a diagnosis than getting the pain under control. I wanted some semblance of a normal, comfortable life back for our son. We tried stronger drugs with more side effects and risks then waited for them to take effect. As mentioned, many arthritis drugs take days or weeks to work at their optimal levels, which means treatment can be frustratingly slow. I was grateful, at least, that we were dealing with all this during winter break, so that missing school and the stress of catching up were not issues.

Miraculously, we found a drug that worked. Slowly but surely, Grant felt a little better with each passing day. By the time six weeks had passed (the amount of time we were told it would take for the drug to be full strength in his system), his pain had almost vanished. We were thrilled. And, for the first time, his rheumatologist believed we were in fact dealing with a form of juvenile arthritis or childhood autoimmune disease. Although his labs had always been normal, his symptoms and the length of time he endured them, along with his response to treatment, all pointed in that direction. We had also ruled out all the common reasons for his problem.

At long last, ten years after the initial onset of symptoms, we had a diagnosis. It was a relief to finally know what was wrong, but we soon learned that having a diagnosis is only the beginning. We had one answer, but a lot more questions.

My Kid Has JA, Now What?

The Big Umbrella

If you're anything like me, you probably knew very little about arthritis in children before the JA diagnosis. That's an old person's problem, right? When most people hear the term *arthritis*, they think of osteoarthritis; the kind your grandparents have; the kind you get after you've lived a long life and worn down your joints. The fact is arthritis in children is often misunderstood as a "pain only" syndrome—something they should be able to get over or grow out of.

However, juvenile arthritis is far bigger. It's actually an umbrella term used to describe the many autoimmune and inflammatory conditions that can develop in children age 16 or younger. The definition of arthritis is joint (*arthro*) inflammation (*itis*), but JA can be much, much more. It can involve the eyes, skin, and gastrointestinal tract. It can be systemic, involving the internal organs, or localized in one or several joints. There are also many types of JA, including juvenile dermatomyositis, scleroderma, lupus, and juvenile spondyloarthropathies. The most common form of JA is juvenile idiopathic arthritis (JIA), historically referred to as juvenile rheumatoid arthritis (JRA). According to the Arthritis Foundation, JIA is defined as swelling in at least one or more joints, lasting at least six weeks. That's why for most it takes *at least* six weeks to diagnose! JIA is further broken down into six categories: oligoarthritis, polyarthritis, systemic, enthesitis-related, psoriatic, and "other," which includes children who exhibit features from two or more types or have symptoms in excess of six weeks that do not meet the criteria of any other form.

So what does all that mean? It means that JA is an umbrella term that covers a multitude of afflictions. It also means that your child's JA diagnosis and treatment plan are probably going to look a lot different than my child's. There are so many different types of juvenile arthritis with diverse symptoms and manifestations that very rarely will two cases look alike. This is probably one of the most important things I can tell you if your child has been newly diagnosed: Do not let yourself get wrapped up in someone else's case, thinking that's what will happen in your family!

We live in the information age, which can be both a blessing and a curse. One of the first things many of us do is perform a Google search to find out all the facts. If you search for juvenile arthritis, you will find some pretty dramatic stories. For every one of these, there are just as many cases that aren't as serious. The things you read about JA and the other children you meet may or may not have things in common with your child.

No Two Cases Are the Same

It could be better, it could be worse, or it could cycle somewhere between the two. The more friends you make in the rheumatology clinic waiting room or the JA community, the more you will find pieces of their experiences that mirror yours. This can provide you with valuable information and support, but it's just another piece of the puzzle. Over time, *you* will become the expert in your child's symptoms, reactions, and responses. Gaining this knowledge, learning as much as you can, and conveying it to your child's healthcare team is what will make the difference in his or her treatment, regardless of the type of JA that has been diagnosed.

Déjà Vu—Well, Not Really

A perfect illustration of how different two cases can be is the story of my two sons. Genetically, they are pretty similar. They have the same parents, they are both boys, and they were born less than two years apart, so many of their experiences and environmental exposures were the same. Just as two children raised similarly in the same family can have completely opposite personalities, the way JA has "shown" itself to each of my boys could not be more different.

Grant's diagnosis took more than ten years to nail down. Even after that determination and treatment, things spiraled out of control and got so much worse. He had a severe allergic reaction to one of the medications (ironically, the only one that was working on his rheumatologic issues) that nearly cost him his life. He developed DRESS syndrome (a type of severe drug reaction), non-viral hepatitis, eosinophilia, and a whole host of other serious issues. He spent time as an inpatient in the hospital and subsequently missed nearly four months of school. In this weakened state, JA took an even greater hold on him, and it felt as though we would never get him back to "normal."

Calculating the Odds

Over the next two years, as I watched him struggle to get back to the life he used to have, I had a new respect for what JA could do and the kind of opponent with which we were dealing. I was also very worried it could happen to my younger son, as well. Even though it is fairly uncommon for siblings to develop JIA (Grant's diagnosis), it was still a concern. Every little ache or pain Evan mentioned seemed like a red flag, and every time he walked off the playing field looking stiff or sore, I wondered if I was overlooking something, just like I had with Grant. I never knew if I was worrying too much, or just making sure I didn't make the same mistakes twice.

Many studies have been done on the subject, and the generally accepted consensus, as reported by the Arthritis Foundation, is that 1 out of every 1,000 children under the age of 16 has JIA. In families where one child has already been diagnosed, the risk of siblings developing JIA could be up to 12 times higher than in the general population and up to six times higher for first cousins. Dr. Sampath Prahalad, a medical doctor and associate professor of Pediatrics and Human Genetics at Emory University, conducted one of these studies and states, "With a population prevalence of JIA at one in 1,000, a 12-time greater risk may sound like a lot but it's only equal to 1.2 percent." That would mean that even a full sibling of a JIA child has a 98.8 percent chance of *not* developing the disease. Knowing these statistics made me feel that watching Evan so closely for signs of JIA was akin to waiting for lightning to strike him while he held a metal bat at baseball practice … it could happen, but probably not.

Grant required so much of my attention and energy at the time that I felt worry was a wasted emotion. Worrying wouldn't fix anything, it wouldn't guarantee that Evan didn't have JA, or get him diagnosed faster if he did. The best I could do was to keep an eye on him, let the doctors observe him more frequently, and have him treated if unexplained symptoms popped up.

When Evan was 11½, just about the same age as Grant when he was diagnosed, I started to notice that he was complaining more about joint pain. Truthfully, learning those odds, being armed with the doctors' assurances, and knowing that his pediatrician was monitoring him made me think there was probably nothing to worry about. His lab work had been fine, his physical exams unremarkable, and his personality, well, that was a factor, too.

Like Night and Day

I love both my children dearly. I often joke that in my life, if Grant is the sugar, Evan is the spice. He is witty, humorous, and definitely a fun guy to be around. Part of what makes him so entertaining is his ability to put himself 110 percent into whatever he is doing or feeling, and along with those characteristics comes a flair for the dramatic. Even as a baby, Evan was the loudest belly-laugher and the biggest wailer—a stubbed toe was nearly equivalent to the end of the world. Most of the time I would get a pretty accurate picture if I took what Evan described and then reduced it by half. That's just Evan. So, you can see why I might take some of his aches and pains with a grain of salt.

The same way I convinced myself that the two-year-old Grant was jealous over his new brother, I convinced myself that Evan just needed some special attention after all my energies had been focused on Grant. He had been seeing the doctor regularly, so I felt all my bases were covered.

Then one night, while I was giving Grant one of his regular injections, Evan came into the room, angry, complaining that he hurt, too. He told me, "Grant isn't the only one dealing with pain every day." He was upset and said he knew I didn't care. He had visited the doctor a few days before with his mystery pains, but we had found nothing. Evan and I had talks from time to time about the difference between JIA pains and everyday annoyances caused by overexertion on the playground or the ball field. While I finished up with Grant, I was getting ready to have "the talk" with Evan again. But, as he turned to walk out of the room, I saw it: Both of his elbows were red and swollen.

I asked him to hold on and tell me more about the pain. Since he was in between sports, did he do something out of the ordinary in gym class? Was something new hurting him? He told me his shoulder and elbows were the problem this time, and that I never wanted to listen. He hadn't "done" anything, but everything still hurt. I felt his elbows and got that sinking feeling in the pit of my stomach. They were swollen with fluid and had that familiar warm feeling of a JA afflicted joint.

It took *three* visits before Evan's elbows were red and swollen at the same time he was at the doctor. Remember how I said JA is sneaky? Sometimes it shows itself and sometimes it doesn't? Well, in this instance, we outsmarted JA. I took pictures of his joints when they were at their worst and kept track of the cycles for the doctors. By April 2012, just a few months after he experienced his first symptoms, Evan was diagnosed with JIA.

At first, I was just sick. I thought I knew what we were in for. We had just been on a wild and crazy ride with Grant's problems, and I was bracing myself for the worst. I had no idea how I would handle *two* children with JIA. Emotionally, how could I bear watching both of them go through it? I felt sorry for myself for a little while, and even sorrier for my sons. Then do you know what I did? I picked myself up and moved on. Worry didn't make a difference before, and I knew it wouldn't make a difference the second time around. But a funny thing happened as I prepared for the worst—nothing ever really happened. Evan's case could not have been more different than Grant's.

Research indicates that with siblings who have JIA, the onset is usually around the same age and of the same subtype. Well, that certainly held true for us: The ages and subtypes were spot-on, but the symptoms and severity were far different. Grant had chronic inflammation and pain, needing a number of daily medications just to control his symptoms. With Evan, every couple of months we might see some swelling, redness, warmth, or increased pain in a joint, at which time we administer medication. In his case, only mild doses of NSAIDs are necessary to head off a flare and then can be discontinued in a few days. Unlike Grant, we also found Evan to be neutropenic (more susceptible to infections), but although it takes him longer to get over a cold or other virus, it doesn't really change his everyday life. JA has not affected his school work, his sleep, or his ability to participate in activities. In fact, other than it just being "out there" for us to think about and treat briefly every now and again, the JA is almost a *non*-factor in Evan's life. Almost, because we still have a healthy respect for what it *can* do and we know the enemy is close. Still, it's hard to believe it's even the same disease!

Developing Your Own Strategies

The sooner you understand how unique your child's case of JA is, the better you will be able to focus on his or her specific issues and facilitate the best possible care and treatments. I want you to skip over the stage where you try to have everything make sense in someone else's frame of reference. I don't want you to buy into the "cousin so-and so's kid had a friend who had JA and they did *xyz* so that's what little Johnny needs, too," or the "I knew someone at work whose kid nearly died from that disease," or the well-meaning neighbor who says "little Jane a few blocks over is supposed to have that, but it's not real in kids, she just fakes it." Don't let yourself go there because none of these scenarios will be completely accurate. JA simply doesn't work that way.

Let me use a sports analogy. In 1972, Don Shula led the Miami Dolphins to the only perfect season in football history. In 2007, the Miami Dolphins only won one game. What happened? It was still the Dolphins. They still had players and coaches. It was still football. The reason why the 2007 team didn't have a perfect season is because they had different players, different coaches, different weather conditions, and different opponents. JA is like the Miami Dolphins. It morphs with the players and the circumstances.

Expecting the same thing from JA for every kid is like expecting the Miami Dolphins to have a perfect season (or not-so-perfect season) *every* year. The 2008 Dolphins improved their season to 11-5 by making adjustments and knowing what they were up against. Every child is a whole other ball game, and when they are diagnosed, it starts a whole new season with a unique set of challenges. I'm here to help you develop *your own* strategies to make it the best season possible.

CHAPTER TWO

The Game Changer

Just when you think you have things figured out, life tends to throw you a curve ball. Juvenile idiopathic arthritis (JIA) has been a game changer for our family. Much the same way many of us define our lives by milestones such as before or after college, marriage, or kids, we now refer to our life in two stages: before and after Grant became ill.

The turning point wasn't the day we received a firm diagnosis, as you might expect, or the rough patches we endured when Grant was up so many nights in pain. For us, the big event that changed our lives forever, forming a concrete division between now and then, was the first inpatient hospital admission for Grant in February 2010. Evan's diagnosis two years later was devastating in its own right, but we were already living out a "new normal," where everything in our lives was framed within the context of JA. Evan's diagnosis was like another game in our new season, whereas Grant's first major hospital admission made us realize we were in a completely different league.

Chain Reaction

In the days leading up to the big event, there were many significant changes in Grant's care. We were working hard to determine what medications could help him finally get some relief. We had changed pediatricians, as recommended by his pediatric rheumatologist, to another great doctor with a little more autoimmune experience. We had exhausted the possibility of other issues causing his pain and inflammation, so we were moving forward from a rheumatology perspective. Our approach was now more focused and deliberate.

We thought everything was progressing in the right direction, albeit slowly, and had no idea what lay ahead. The chain of events triggered by Grant's reaction to the latest medication changed everything, not just for Grant, but for our entire family. The hospital visit was the catalyst to it all.

Grant had started complaining of nausea, which can be expected with many rheumatology medications. Even though his pain was exponentially better, he started to resist the idea of taking his medication because it made him feel so awful. After a few weeks, we noticed he was developing a strange rash, which resembled sandpaper, on his torso. Things just deteriorated from there. In a matter of days, he was unable to keep down food or liquids, and the sandpaper rash was evolving into bigger, very red bumps. After consulting with the doctor, we decided to withhold his medications, just in case he was having a strange side effect. Honestly, we didn't think the medication was the culprit since he had been on it without issues for over a month, but we were coming up on a weekend and thought it would be better safe than sorry.

Have you ever noticed that kids seem to get their sickest at the *worst* possible times? Usually on the weekend or the middle of the night, when the doctors aren't available? Well, that's exactly what happened. It was Super Bowl Sunday—a big deal in our house, since not only are my guys avid sports fans, but we also typically know someone who is playing in the game every year! The first huge warning sign that something was very wrong was that Grant was too sick to watch the game, fading in and out of sleep. This was so out of character for him. He had also vomited multiple times, and his lips were starting to become parched and cracked. No matter what I tried to give him—hot drinks, cold beverages, or even ice chips—I couldn't get him to keep any fluids down. As the day wore on, he started running a fever and became more lethargic. I was getting very concerned, but short of the going to the ER, what could I do on a Sunday? I thought if we could just hold out until the morning, we would squeeze into the doctor's office again.

Then came the straw that broke the camel's back: Grant wanted to go to the restroom, but was unable to get there on his own, or urinate when he got there. He was too weak and dehydrated. When I looked at his torso, I saw that the rash was spreading and there was no "white" to be seen. In a matter of just a few hours, he went from appearing "rashy" to looking like he had been scrubbed with a cheese grater. Because his condition had gone downhill at such an alarming rate, I knew I didn't have another night to spare. So, I grabbed a couple of things and we headed to the emergency room at the children's hospital.

The Tip of the Iceberg

Amazingly, we had only been to the ER with Grant once before. We were always that lucky family that never had anything so catastrophic that it warranted an emergency room visit. Somehow we had always managed to wait for normal business hours to see our regular doctors. The one incident that required an ER visit was the time Grant's rheumatologist wanted us to bring him in for STAT blood work during an especially bad flare. (Remember how I said kids always get sick at the *worst* times? Well, that happened over a three-day weekend!) Due to my inexperience with the ER, I was surprised at how long it took to get any treatment. It was crowded, and since Grant wasn't actively bleeding and there were no bones protruding from his body, we had to wait.

One of the things I have learned about *all* autoimmune diseases, including JA, is that things can look fairly good on the outside, but tell a completely different story on the inside. Often what you see is just the tip of the iceberg. By the time we were seen by a doctor, the only unaffected skin on Grant's body was a sliver the size of an almond under his chin. Even then, I naively thought he would get some type of IV drugs to help with the reaction, as well as to rehydrate him, and then we would go home to ride it out. Unfortunately, the nightmare was just beginning.

Since we were at a teaching hospital, the ER had a number of residents who saw Grant before he was examined by a regular staff doctor. New doctors, coupled with an environment that is more suited to trauma than complicated medical histories, further delayed treatment. At one point, Grant started having difficulty breathing, which escalated the situation. When the attending physician finally came in, he took one look at him and informed us that Grant would be admitted to the hospital that evening and reevaluated for release the next day.

One day turned into two, and two turned into seven. After a brief two-day respite at home, Grant was readmitted to the hospital for a total stay of ten days. Early in our stay, two residents came into Grant's room in the middle of the night when they thought we were sleeping. As they performed the normal vital checks, I overheard them speaking in hushed tones; they said Grant was a very sick young man and gave him a 50-50 chance of "making it." I couldn't believe what I was hearing! The JIA, along with the medications, had started a domino effect of serious conditions, including non-viral hepatitis and DRESS (Drug Reaction with Eosinophilia and Systemic Symptoms) syndrome. To my horror, the possibility of Stevens-Johnson syndrome (a life-threatening skin condition) and potential liver failure was mentioned several times.

Without warning, everything had been turned upside down—and it changed all of us. Grant's battle for survival altered our lives irrevocably. Everything that happened from this hospital admission on has become our "new normal," a completely different life than we had before.

Although Grant's condition improved and he was eventually released from the hospital, he was still very sick. As a condition of our release, Grant had blood draws every other day to monitor his liver. Our new life was filled with regular hospital visits and admissions, frequent lab work, multiple therapies, medications, and doctors' appointments. There was very little room in the schedule for school, and most of the time, he was too weak or sick to go anyway. We had gone from seeing our son play football and recover from the exertion in a day or two to barely walking unassisted and struggling for his life in a span of just three months. The changes were huge, and they weren't restricted to just Grant … everything was different.

HOSPITAL TIPS

I won't lie: a week in the hospital feels like a month. However, there are some things you can do to make your hospital stay a little easier.

Pack Light, But Smart. There is next to no space for anything personal, especially luggage, so just bring a small duffel bag. Depending on the procedures and the hospital, your child may be able to wear their own pajamas, but you will still need something that offers easy access to their chest for exams and their arms for IVs. Make sure it's not a favorite pair of pj's, as there is always a chance of stains. Always have an extra pair on hand in case he or she has an accident (accidental urination is a common side effect of steroids) and needs to change clothes. For yourself, make sure you have regular clothes you can easily sleep in and not look overly rumpled the next morning. I had a couple of cute velour track suits that fit the bill. Leggings and a big cotton sweater or shirt are also good bets. You may be up every two hours or so during the night, and there are lots of people running in and out at all hours, so pajamas aren't really practical. Make sure to bring flip-flops (shower shoes) in case you get a chance to use the parent shower. They are also convenient to slip on when you have to pop out of your chair to get something for your child. Make sure your child also has slippers (a big improvement over the ugly hospital "grippy" socks). You can be barefoot in bed, but must have your feet covered out of bed.

Pack a Spare Bag to Leave at Home. When you need new clothes, having a bag already packed makes it easier for the other parent or helpful relative/friend to swap bags, and then wash and replace what was in the old bag for the next go-around. Be sure to include some snacks (see below).

HOSPITAL TIPS

Bring Food for *You!* Let's face it, the food options at most hospitals leave much to be desired and can be expensive. Since the staff must monitor the calorie intake for patients, nibbling on your child's leftovers is not an option. Bringing your own snacks is the best bet. And since beverage machines aren't always conveniently located, I started bringing a lunchbox-sized soft-sided cooler: I would buy several drinks at a time and keep the extras in the room. Having your own food and drinks is also handy when you're hungry or thirsty in the middle of the night. Check with the hospital before bringing anything with nuts, due to allergies. Also, having gum or mints is a good idea, especially when the doctor wants to talk to you at 3:00 a.m.!

Take a Pen and Notepad. Write *everything* down—you will thank me later. Whenever they put something in the IV, ask what it is and when it will be needed next. Write it down and note the time, plus the time it will be needed again. With painkillers, it's very important not to lapse for the first couple days; it's hard to get back to a good spot if they run out. The nurses are overworked and will sometimes run late. If they say 4–6 hours, buzz them and remind them at hour five, which allows plenty of time to requisition the pharmacy and work your child into their regular rounds. Writing information down is also a good way to catch errors; the staff is only human and has many patients. You only have *one* patient to track. I have caught errors this way, and most of the other parents I have spoken with concur. Additionally, if you write everything down, you won't have to ask the same questions over and over. You will receive *a lot* of information, and eventually it all starts to blend together. If you write it down, you can revisit it. Also, jot down your questions for the doctor

HOSPITAL TIPS

when you think of them. Believe me, you'll have a long list of questions in middle of the night and won't remember a single one when the doctor arrives for his morning rounds!

Bring Headphones and Other Gadgets. Headphones can be a lifesaver for both you and your child. If your child has a roommate who cries or screams (as many younger patients do), it can be very unnerving. We passed the time watching movies on my laptop and using our iPods. We also watched an entire television series on DVD (a series can really make the time fly by). The hospital television does no good if your child's roommate is having visitors or watching something else. If your child is old enough, you may consider allowing them to have a Facebook account so they can keep in touch with friends. For Grant, this was a social lifeline! He could chat with friends in real time, and I was there to supervise. Also, keep in mind that if you have a young child in the room, the nurses will turn off the room lights early, so bring a book light if you plan to read.

Bring a Pillowcase and Blanket. Hospital linens are typically scratchy. And besides, a colorful pillowcase from home is much more cheery. It's amazing how such a small comfort can make such a big difference. You will also need your own pillow, and both you and your child will want a twin-size blanket or throw. I prefer fleece because it's warm and washes up easily. Sure, the hospital has blankets but, again, they are usually thin and scratchy, and sometimes the only thing they provide parents is a sheet. After a few days, this little added comfort will make your stay ten times better. Of course, don't bring anything too expensive or that your child loves, because there's a good chance it will get stained.

Rest. I realize it's easier said than done, but rest whenever you can—

HOSPITAL TIPS

and don't feel guilty or indulgent. Schedules are crazy in the hospital, so if you can catch a catnap at the same time as your child, you should. Vital checks, routine monitoring, and medication administration make it hard to snooze more than an hour or two at any time, night or day, and sleep will help give you the mental clarity you need to communicate with the doctors. This small attempt at taking care of yourself is actually an important part of ensuring your child will get the best possible care.

Plan Ahead. Depending on the admission (anticipated for a procedure or an emergency that results in inpatient stay), you may have a few days or just an hour or two to prepare. After our first admission, I had a bag packed and ready to go for each of us, just in case, and kept the "right" snacks stocked in our home so I wasn't making an extra trip to the store.

Don't Be Afraid to Ask. Once you're at the hospital, ask the nurse if she will order the thick pads that resemble egg crates for your chair and your child's bed. They are usually available, but you have to ask. After getting settled, ask your assigned nurse what other services are available. For instance, do they allow you to check out video game consoles? Do they have DVDs on loan? At children's hospitals, they usually have a child life activity center, as well as child life specialists who can bring age-appropriate diversions to your child when he or she is feeling well enough.

Don't Bring Too Many Activities. It may seem counterintuitive, but if you supply every imaginable activity to keep your child occupied, there won't be anything left for visitors to bring. When friends and relatives ask what to bring, you can recommend activities that your child enjoys, such as crossword puzzles, Sudoku, crafts, or books. This way, your child will feel loved and surprised, and the activities will be spread throughout their stay.

The New Normal

The upheaval we experienced from Grant's illness spread to all areas of our lives and affected the entire family. Evan no longer had the "homeroom mom" he did before. Caring for Grant and making doctors' appointments had priority over bake sales and field trips. I saw Evan very little during this period, even though I was still a stay-at-home mom. Thankfully, Grandma helped with homework and picked him up from school while his dad was still at work. Time with my husband also diminished—we rarely even slept in the same room, since he needed to rest for work, and I was up to give Grant his medications every couple of hours. The schedule was almost like having a newborn again.

Because Grant's immune system was so suppressed due to the medications, we no longer had friends over to the house. We had been warned about exposing him to others who could possibly be ill or carriers of illness. We thought twice about going out for anything but the necessities for the same reason. It felt as though we had become prisoners in our own home.

Nothing was routine anymore, and we all had to adjust. Most parenting websites and books will tell you that children *need* routines. Even when dealing with a chronic illness (some would say even more so), it's important to stick to as many daily routines and habits as possible in order to help the child cope with his or her new reality. While I agree with this advice, I learned it doesn't always work. When there is a flare or a big bump in the road, such as a hospital stay, everything goes out the window! There is no routine. You deal with things as they come.

With many other illnesses, there are defined beginnings and endings, courses of actions and expected outcomes. The autoimmune family of conditions is far less predictable. Just when you think you have a good rhythm going with medication or have established the right balance between rest and activities, something changes, and your child may respond differently each time. It will take time to figure out what works best for your child and your family. Then whatever you found to be "best" will evolve. Being adamant about sticking to one plan or routine that *did* work will just drive yourself (and others around you) insane! It can be very disconcerting, but there are things you can do to ease the transitions.

MOVING THROUGH THE STAGES OF GRIEF

In many ways, being diagnosed with a chronic illness or having someone you love being diagnosed with one is a death of sorts. Even though the prognosis may be good, it's the end of the "old" life as you knew it and the beginning of a new, sometimes dramatically different life. In her 1969 work *Death and Dying*, renowned sociologist Elisabeth Kübler-Ross defined five stages of grief. Although the original intent was related to the feelings faced at the end of life, I believe most parents will see themselves in the model she outlined. The following are my interpretations of the Kübler-Ross stages of grief as they apply to your child being diagnosed with a chronic illness.

Denial—In this stage you don't want to believe this is your child's diagnosis. You may think the doctors are wrong, the test results are off, or simply that your child will be one of the first to "grow out of it," his or her symptoms magically disappearing the same way they appeared. Regardless, you're not ready to admit that your child may have a serious, incurable condition.

Anger—After the realization hits that your child does in fact have the condition, anger sets in. *Why did this have to happen to us? Why him/her?* This anger can be manifested in many different ways, toward oneself, toward others, or even God.

Bargaining—Many times the bargaining stage involves offers to a higher power—*"if only x will change, I will do y."* It's a natural way of coping; an attempt to gain some control over a situation that seems devoid of control.

Depression—This is the time when we truly grieve for what has been lost. Feelings of regret, fear, and even hopelessness are common as the reality of the situation sets in. Being depressed is a natural part of the process, but you can't let yourself stay there.

Acceptance—At this stage some of the emotion is removed and is replaced by practicality. The reality of the diagnosis is accepted, and you begin to form plans and take action. Your focus becomes: *"What do we need to do to make our child feel better?"* You also learn to make the best of the situation.

Flexibility Is Key

I used to have a fairly fixed schedule. Bedtime was bedtime; breakfast was an hour before we left for school; and so on. We had rules, and we stuck to them. For instance, if you were too sick to go to school, then you were too sick to attend a party after school, end of discussion. All that changed after my children's JIA diagnoses. Although we try hard not to let JA be a crutch for skipping out on responsibilities, we have learned that some rules need to be reevaluated based on the circumstances. Flexibility is the key. It's the only way to balance the needs of the whole child and the whole family, while preserving your sanity.

Take after-school events, for example. After several weeks of homebound instruction, Grant was invited to play video games at a friend's house with a few other boys. The mom was aware of his issues and invited me to stay for coffee while the boys socialized. Grant was still in too much pain to attend even a half day of school, let alone be exposed to so many germs, but he was missing *real* human interaction with kids his own age. Despite the fact that his teacher didn't come that day (he was ill from a methotrexate injection, a common chemo drug also used for rheumatology patients), I allowed Grant to visit with his friends. He was feeling better by the afternoon, none of the boys were sick, and he *needed* that time. I was able to be there in case we had to cut the visit short, and it was a very brief visit by design. Just a few months before, I never would have agreed: He didn't do his "work," therefore he didn't earn his "play." Those were the old rules, and in our old life, they were good ones! Now, however, rigidly following that rule would prevent Grant from socializing, ever. To complicate matters further, the times when Grant was feeling good didn't necessarily correspond with the times his friends were free (or free of sniffles!), so coordinating a date when all the appropriate conditions were met would be nearly impossible.

Unfortunately, some parents didn't understand how Grant could be receiving homebound services, be too ill to go to school, and yet be well enough to attend a birthday party, even if it was for just an hour on the weekend. If I didn't jump on every opportunity when Grant felt well enough to socialize, he would never be able to attend. Stringently abiding by the rules was less important than preserving the tiny glimpses of joy and friendship in his life. Being flexible helped us to find that balance.

Different Priorities

Although our lives had changed dramatically, and we desperately wanted "the old Grant" back, JA did not define our lives. If anything, it created a paradigm shift in our family. It gave us a newfound appreciation of our old life, and life, period. We learned not to take any day for granted, and we reveled in the small successes. Sleeping through the night, going to school, even for a few hours, walking … things previously overlooked as givens were now cause for celebration.

We developed thicker skins, but at the same time expanded our empathy for others. We had witnessed, firsthand, so much suffering and sorrow. During Grant's hospital stay, one of the other children on our floor lost their battle. We had met the family in the break room and talked together over coffee. We also heard the crash cart barreling down the hall in the middle of the night and saw the anguish when there was nothing left for the staff to do. This illness suddenly became *very* real. Hearing of another seriously or chronically ill child hits much closer to home now; and it still creates some very raw emotions, especially for Grant, who, at the tender age of eleven, was faced with his own mortality for the very first time.

At face value, this may all seem very depressing—truthfully, it *was* a very sad and difficult time. But that is only half the story. Although I would never choose this for my child, it has made our family stronger. It has made Grant stronger. We laugh harder and, of course, cry harder, too. In some ways, we feel much more alive! We have also become more grateful than ever—for Grant being a fighter, for friends and family who have come through for us, and for the simplest of joys. By necessity, we have streamlined our life and, in the process, reevaluated our priorities. We have found support in the most unlikely places and renewed our faith. Although the situation we experienced was quite a challenge (and still is, but on a much lesser scale), I am reminded that the only way coal becomes a diamond is through heat and pressure, squeezing out the impurities to create something even better. How you approach this disease will make a difference in how it affects your family. We didn't choose JA, but we can choose how to live with it. We've decided to let it change us for the better, and so can you.

CHAPTER THREE

An Unpredictable Opponent

Did you know that juvenile arthritis is one of the most common childhood diseases in the United States? Approximately 300,000 American children are affected by pediatric arthritis and rheumatologic conditions—and the numbers are on the rise. And, yet, there is a great deal that is still unknown about this affliction. As I touched on earlier, there is no set course of treatment; symptoms can vary widely from child to child; and even the diagnosis can change over time since there are so many forms of the disease. It's unpredictable, to say the least.

The broadest definition of juvenile arthritis is any form of arthritis or arthritis-related condition that develops in children or teens younger than the age of 16. The most common form is juvenile idiopathic arthritis (JIA), which means "from unknown cause." Unlike osteoarthritis (the type you associate with aging and overuse of joints), juvenile arthritis (JA) is usually an autoimmune disorder. In adults, the condition is referred to as rheumatoid arthritis (RA). In both cases, the immune system attacks some of the body's healthy cells and tissues. Research suggests that it may be a two-step process: something in the genes (a genetic predisposition or the presence of a known marker such as HLA-B27) makes the body more conducive to the development of the condition, and then something else, like a virus, can set it off.

The way an attack is manifested depends on the type of JA the child has.

Once the child is diagnosed, the next challenge is to determine the specific type. The first six months after diagnosis are especially important, because each type of JA can respond to treatments and medications differently. In fact, certain treatments are only used for some subtypes and not for others. However, during an episode of high inflammation or "flare," some treatments, such as the use of steroids, are common across all types. To further confuse matters, some children respond better to medications that are *atypical* treatments for their type. For example, our son Grant responded better to some medications used for juvenile dermatomyositis (JDM) than those typically used for his first diagnosis of enthesitis-related JIA, despite the absence of a JDM diagnosis! The earlier the specific type is determined, the better chance the medical team has to limit or even reverse possible damage to the parts of the body that are under attack.

The Big Picture

In the beginning, I just wanted a firm diagnosis. When the doctors felt that it was enthesitis-related JIA, I thought, "Okay, now we can make a plan." But that diagnosis morphed into probable spondyloarthropathy because Grant was showing signs of bowel disease (a condition that is commonly related to spondyloarthropathy). So, we mentally shifted gears. From there, we heard rumblings of systemic arthritis, psoriatic arthritis, urticaria, autoimmune diabetes, episcleritis, and uveitis, to name a few medical conditions. Some of the symptoms related to these other conditions materialized, while others didn't. Certain symptoms seemed to appear out of the blue, each requiring the opinion of a specialist. As a matter of fact, our son was collecting specialists faster than a 12-year-old boy collects baseball cards! He was seen by doctors in rheumatology, allergy, hematology/oncology, infectious disease, immunology, orthopedic surgery, dermatology, gastroenterology, cardiology, ophthalmology, endocrinology, neurology, psychology, pain management, and ear, nose and throat! It was overwhelming.

Eventually, I learned to focus less on the specific diagnoses (that is the doctor's job) and more on getting Grant the treatment he needed. Worrying about this syndrome or that subtype changed nothing. Simply put, no matter how we decided to define it to the world, his body was attacking itself. In the beginning, the where, when, and how seemed to change with the direction of the wind. My job was to help the doctors pin down what was going on when they *couldn't* observe him, and then help get him the right treatments and the right care at the right time. In comparison, my younger son Evan's case has been much less complicated, involving a few issues that have been easily managed on the first attempt, with just a couple of doctors in the mix. Like I said, every case is different.

Educate to Communicate

Nevertheless, educating yourself about the different types of pediatric autoimmune conditions can be helpful to communicate with the doctors. One of the best resources I have found is Dr. Thomas Lehman's book *It's Not Just Growing Pains*, which covers all types of JA and related conditions. Keep in mind, there can be quite a bit of overlap from one type to the next, so just because you may see similar symptoms don't panic and don't self-diagnose! Use that information to help the doctor.

As an example, lupus runs in our family, and many of Grant's symptoms (after his first hospital discharge) seemed to mirror cases of lupus that I had researched. Grant did *not* have lupus, but framing his symptoms in a context that was well known to the doctor helped me effectively communicate what was happening to Grant on a cyclical basis. Doing research, reading books authored by recognized experts, and familiarizing myself with other cases gave me the tools I needed to better convey my child's situation. Using terms and contexts common to autoimmune disease put me on the same page as the doctors, and we started speaking more of the same language.

Know Your Adversary

Battling an unpredictable opponent is tough. It's difficult to make a game plan and stick to it. As the enemy changes, so must the plan! One of the best ways to prepare is to learn as much as possible so that you can be ready for any situation. When my husband coached youth and high school football, one of the ways he prepared his team for upcoming games was to watch film taken of the opponent. He didn't just watch the prior week's game; he watched all the film he could get his hands on. He observed how they handled each of *their* opponents, because each game was different.

Juvenile arthritis is different in every child. By observing how other kids act and react to JA, it can give you snippets of the opponent *your* child will face in his or her battle. Reading about their lives and their struggles is like watching game film for your child. It may not be your particular game, but it shows you what that opponent is capable of and how to prepare against it.

Meet Some of the Other Players

The following are actual accounts shared by families living with different types of JA. Their stories illustrate how diverse the paths to diagnosis and treatment can be, as well as the unpredictable nature of this disease. However, while their stories are different, there is a common thread—hope.

Connor's Journey with JDM by Anke

In 2005, my husband and I were thrilled to become parents by adopting one-year-old identical twin boys from Russia. The adoption of our boys was such a gift, and they have brought us immeasurable joy, despite the medical challenges we've faced. Because our sons were adopted from a foreign country, we did not receive any medical history on the boys or their parents. As we soon learned, this lack of information can make diagnosing health problems more difficult.

Shortly after we arrived home with our sons, the "younger" twin, Alexander, was diagnosed with a tethered spinal cord, which required corrective surgery when he was just 18 months old. He had a dimple on his back that led to this diagnosis, but his brother, Connor, had no outward signs of the condition. However, a few months later, as I was watching a documentary on syndromes that can develop during pregnancy, a warning bell went off in my head.

Since our boys were identical twins, I took Connor in for an assessment. Sure enough, an MRI revealed he also had a tethered spinal cord. Like his brother, he underwent surgery shortly after he turned two. Though the surgeries were stressful, we thought the worst was behind us.

In 2009, as we were preparing for our yearly trip to Germany (where I was born and raised), warnings about the swine flu filled the news. We were told it was even more widespread in Europe and, as a precaution, the boys should receive the H1N1 flu shot. They were vaccinated about three days before our flight, and while we were in the airport Connor started complaining about pain in his legs. We brushed it off as growing pains or the normal aches of a very active five-year-old.

However, during our stay in Germany the pain got progressively worse. I was so concerned that I changed our travel plans to come home early. During the return trip, Connor's legs were so sore that I had to carry him most of the time. Our first stop upon arrival home was the doctor's office.

The first diagnosis we received was mononucleosis. We were told to take him home and give him Motrin for the discomfort. But, Connor did not get better. In fact, his condition worsened, and that's when the "Mommy Bear" instinct kicked in. I took him back to the doctor *three* more times, until finally a physician's assistant put me in touch with a neurologist.

Initially, we were worried about a reattachment of the spinal cord, but the MRI came back clear. The next step was a spinal tap to rule out Guillain-Barré syndrome, which can occur after receiving a vaccination. When this test came back negative, Connor had a muscle biopsy done, which confirmed that his muscles were inflamed and he was put on a steroid. We had to wait weeks for the complete results, but in January 2011, we were told that our son had juvenile dermatomyositis (JDM), a rare form of juvenile arthritis. More specifically, JDM is a systemic autoimmune disease that causes inflamed and weakened muscles, among other things.

We had a diagnosis, but we did not have the answers we needed to make Connor better. The steroids didn't make a dent in his condition, and Connor declined at a rapid pace. Taking matters into my own hands, I began to research this disease. My husband and I agreed that we would take Connor anywhere in the world to find the help he needed.

I have to admit, the more I learned about JDM, the more fearful I became. But, then I found a ray of hope: the leading doctor for JDM, Dr. Lauren Pachman, was not a world away but working at The Children's Memorial Hospital in Chicago. I e-mailed her immediately. By this time, Connor was unable to move. He could not walk or lift his arms to feed himself. He would choke when given food and cried when he was touched due to his inflamed muscles. So, you can imagine how relieved I was to get a response to my e-mail within fifteen minutes!

Dr. Pachman told us that Connor must be admitted to a hospital as soon as possible. We packed in haste and flew to Chicago that same afternoon. Little did we know we wouldn't see our home again for almost eight weeks.

After Connor's long hospital stay, his condition improved. He still needs regular physical therapy and lots of medications to keep him stable, but he's doing much better.

While I'm comforted by the fact that we did everything in our power to save Connor's life and get him the treatment he needs, I feel guilty that so much of my focus went toward Connor and not equally on Alexander. I can recall many times when Alexander felt left out as cards and gifts arrived for his brother, while he spent long hours in waiting rooms.

Looking back, I realize that the more Connor was unable to move, the more Alexander moved! A huge part of why Connor fought back so hard against JDM was the fact that his brother motivated him. Like most twins, the boys are very close and share similar traits. As a result, we were invited to be part of a Twin Research Study at the National Institutes of Health in Washington, DC. We are very interested to learn about the possible genetic links regarding JDM, as well as the role of environmental factors. Of course, if JDM is genetic, we worry about what (if anything) may trigger JDM in Alexander.

For now, we are just dreaming of remission or, better yet, a cure! Our boys are now almost nine years old and have found art and painting a great way to express their thoughts and emotions. While it makes me sad to think of the many challenges they have both faced in their young lives, I am also proud of and inspired by their strength.

Dreaming of Running by Lori

Our son, Noah, was a typical nine-year-old boy who loved playing sports of all kinds. Even as a toddler, he showed extraordinary balance and seemed to excel at every activity he attempted. Among his talents was a natural ability to shoot a basketball, and, eventually, he chose that as his main sport. Noah loved playing basketball and people loved to watch him play.

One day, as I watched my son on the basketball court, I noticed he was running "funny" and seemed to be moving slower than usual. After the game, Noah mentioned that his hip was bothering him, which would account for his awkward gait. I chalked it up to him being very active, along with growing pains. However, as the weeks went by, his pain did not subside, so I took him to the pediatrician, who concurred that it was growing pains coupled with activity.

Over the next two years, Noah's symptoms were mild and intermittent. He was still able to play sports, but not nearly with the intensity he once did. At the age of 12, he began complaining of knee and ankle pain and told me his hip was hurting more than usual. I became very concerned when I noticed his knee and ankle were swollen, but again, the pediatrician told us she thought it was due to Noah's rigorous sporting activity and diagnosed a ligament injury. The doctor wrapped his swollen ankle, gave him crutches, and told Noah to stay off it for a while.

Initially, this seemed to work: The swelling went down and the pain improved. I thought he was getting better. Then one evening Noah returned home from a bike ride and could hardly walk. I remember watching him struggle to take each step. He looked at me and said, "Mom, there is something seriously wrong with me. I can't even walk and I'm hurting all over." When I looked down, I could see that both his feet were swollen. That's when I felt the first twinges of panic.

This time I was unwilling to accept the diagnosis of a sports injury, and I pushed the doctor for further testing, which included blood work and an MRI of his knee. Meanwhile, Noah had begun to dread mornings. He was waking up so stiff that he could barely move. He had to rub his hips, knees, ankles, and feet with Mentholatum cream just to get going. I remember dropping him off at school and watching him walk gingerly into the building. His gym class was first on the schedule, and he could not participate in any activities. It was heartbreaking to see him standing on the sidelines.

When I picked him up at the end of the day, his muscles seemed looser and he could move with more ease. Thankfully, he was still able to play on his travel basketball team, but he had trouble running due to his sore feet. As you can imagine, we were confused and frustrated!

At last the doctor called with Noah's test results. His blood work showed an elevated sedimentation (sed) rate and anemia; but honestly, she didn't seem very concerned. She thought the elevated sed rate was the result of a virus and suggested the anemia may be due to poor nutrition. Neither of these explanations sat well with me because Noah had not been sick and he ate a fairly well-rounded diet. However, I took her advice and began giving him vitamins and iron supplements. It wasn't until the results of the MRI came back that the doctor became noticeably concerned. In addition to inflammation, Noah had three unidentified nodules on the back of his knee. We were immediately referred to both an orthopedist and a pediatric oncologist.

The thought of seeing an oncologist was extremely stressful. You see, I was just getting over treatment for an early diagnosis of breast cancer, and the idea of my son going down that road was unbearable. But one step at a time … the orthopedist examined Noah's MRI and seemed baffled. He asked a trusted colleague for a second opinion, who told him the nodules were swollen lymph nodes and suggested we see a pediatric rheumatologist. The combination of inflammation, elevated sed rate, and anemia suggested a rheumatologic condition. Finally, I felt as though we might be getting some long-awaited answers.

Before we had a chance to see the oncologist, he called to say he agreed that the nodules were swollen lymph nodes. I breathed a sigh of relief, but there was still a great deal of uncertainty as to what the rheumatologist would find. Our feelings of apprehension were alleviated somewhat by the warm greeting and comforting words of this doctor. She looked at us and said, "I'm glad you're here, because we're going to help Noah feel better." At long last, words of hope.

All the pieces of the puzzle came together at that appointment. Noah's elevated sed rate was due to active inflammation. The lymph nodes were trying to rid the body of the inflammation, which is why they were swollen. Within minutes, the rheumatologist told us Noah had juvenile enthesitis-related arthritis, which causes pain, swelling, stiffness, and loss of motion in the joints. Enthesitis refers to swelling or inflammation where the tendons or ligaments attach to the bone. We also learned this type of JA affects boys more than girls. In Noah's case, the arthritis was present in his wrists, fingers, one elbow, both his hips, knees, ankles, feet, and even his toes. The good news, the doctor assured us, is that this disease is treatable.

I remember walking out of that office feeling like I could breathe for the first time in months. Though the diagnosis was difficult to hear, my husband and I felt confident we were finally at the right place to get Noah the help he needed. Of course, when it comes to treating JA, there are many different approaches. We started with injections of methotrexate, which is a drug used for chemotherapy. When used in small doses it has been shown to help slow down the immune system from attacking itself—which is what arthritis does. Noah did not like the idea of needles, but was willing to do whatever it took to feel better. Unfortunately, after eight weeks, it was determined this particular drug was not improving Noah's condition.

Our second course of treatment involved steroid injections, which were very painful for Noah, but again, he was such a trooper. And it seemed to work. I remember sending the doctor a message that said, "My son is RUNNING down the hall!" It felt like a miracle—for about two weeks. When the pain and stiffness returned, we all became very discouraged. In addition, the inflammation had begun to affect Noah's growth.

Trial and error are par for the course when it comes to treatment, so we tried a new path. Noah was given an anti-inflammatory along with a biologic drug. It involves a weekly injection, and because it suppresses the immune system, he has a greater chance of developing infection. Another side effect is the increased potential to develop cancer. While the side effects are scary, we decided that getting our active, happy boy back was worth the potential risks. Two weeks after he began the injections, Noah was waking up without stiffness and able to play basketball again. After six weeks, his sed rate had dropped and he actually grew two inches!

In July 2012, the doctor put him into official remission status, which meant he no longer had signs of active disease. If we can go two years without any symptoms (flares), she would start scaling back the medication. She also referred Noah to a physical therapist to work on his range of motion, strength, and balance. In September 2012, Noah ran his first 5K Mud Run.

At the height of his pain, Noah would sometimes wake up and tell me he had dreamed of running. I assured him that he would be able to run again one day, but I had no idea when. To see him active again is truly a blessing. There are times when Noah forgets he has JA, and other times when pain and stiffness are reminders. We have to be very diligent about good hygiene and preventing illness due to his suppressed immune system. But for now, we remain hopeful and confident that we have the right doctor to keep us on track.

Freeing Zoe by Natalie

Confronting my child's illness, one that is confusing and forever changing, in a language that is not my own, has been the most difficult experience in my life. Our daughter Zoe has always been a bit fragile. She suffered continuously with sinus infections since birth. Moreover, she wasn't growing at a "normal" rate. Since all my children were small, I really didn't worry too much when the doctor told me he wasn't happy with her weight gain. I breastfed her and thought maybe the weight charts were based on bottle-fed babies. However, she was classified as "failure to thrive," and I was instructed to introduce certain formulas to her diet, which I did, without much improvement.

After Zoe received her one-year vaccinations, she became very sick. Her temperature soared, and she was lethargic and had diarrhea for four days. We put it down to a reaction to the vaccine and didn't think any more about it.

We were living in France, and the following month we were heading off to Australia to visit family. At 14 months old, Zoe had finally started walking. But, within a week, she suddenly stopped. To be honest, I thought perhaps she was just being lazy. However, three weeks later, as we arrived back home, Zoe was no longer standing up or even crawling. If she wanted to move around, she would slide on her backside or stomach. She had also begun to spike fevers in the afternoon, which would subside after a few hours. Most concerning was her inability to sleep: She would wake up crying six or seven times each night. Once I changed her position, she would fall back asleep.

By the end of August things had gone from bad to worse. Zoe was crying continuously, hardly eating or sleeping, and was extremely fatigued. She would bend up her legs and scream whenever we changed her. Unfortunately, our pediatrician had recently retired, so I took her to see my husband's doctor. He listened to my complaints, weighed her, listened to her chest, and said "She looks fine. If she isn't walking in a month come back and see me." I walked out of there thinking he didn't take me seriously.

Three days later, my husband had his day off and as Zoe lay there, immobile, I pointed to her and said, "Look at her; she isn't moving because she *can't*, not because she doesn't want to!" Filled with concern and frustration, I asked my husband to come back to the doctor with us. This time the doctor seemed to take us seriously. He gave us a referral for an X-ray and an ultrasound for her hips, both of which revealed nothing. The doctor assured us Zoe was fine.

A few days later we ran into Zoe's old pediatrician at the market and spoke to her about what had been happening. Her reaction was much different. She told us to leave the shopping and pack a bag because we needed to go to the hospital now.

Six weeks after the initial doctor's visit, Zoe was finally admitted to the hospital. By this time, she was unable to physically move by herself. I refer to this time as Zoe's "stuck period." In addition to being very sick, she seemed to be trapped inside her own body, and all I wanted to do was set her free.

After numerous tests, the head of pediatrics told us he thought Zoe had a form of juvenile arthritis, but in order to confirm the diagnosis she would need to go to a hospital for rare diseases for children in Paris. In the meantime, they prescribed ibuprofen four times a day. It took another six weeks to receive the final diagnosis—systemic onset juvenile idiopathic arthritis. We learned that her ankles, knees, hips, wrists, elbows, shoulders, lower back, and neck were involved. We also learned that she had inflammation in her liver, lungs, and spleen, which was also affecting her blood.

Trying to sort through what I was being told, translate it into my own words in English, and then understand it was overwhelming. At that point, I just wanted to get on the next plane and take my baby home, where I could make sense of the situation and perhaps feel more in control. After all, knowledge is power ... or so I thought. The reality is this disease is so complex that even if I was being told in English, French, or Chinese, I would still not fully comprehended the implications. How could my baby be given a life-changing diagnosis? How can any parent comprehend the fact that their child will experience chronic pain every day for quite possibly the rest of her life?

Since there is no cure, our focus turned to treatment and pain management. We learned to give our daughter a daily injection, which was as painful as a wasp's sting. Zoe was just 17 months old when we started that treatment—and only 19 months old when the treatment failed.

The next course of treatment involved admission to the hospital for a biweekly infusion. Additionally, for the next two years, Zoe had five days of physiotherapy and hydrotherapy each week. She is now down to two days a week. However, thanks to this treatment, she is now walking, running, and jumping like other three-year-olds.

Of course, it's not always smooth sailing. Zoe is often sick due to her immune system being suppressed (a side effect of the treatment), and recently we have found that her medication is not working as well as it should be. I have learned to take one day at a time and be grateful she can now move around with less pain. Her spirit shines bright and we remain hopeful.

From Head to Toe (Cameron's Story) by Angela

It was August 2009, and our son, Cameron, had just started the third grade. Since it's not uncommon for kids this age to "share" a variety of illnesses, I wasn't particularly worried when I noticed a red, itchy spot on his scalp. The pediatrician took one look at it and diagnosed ringworm. We went home with some nasty-smelling medication, which we finished without improvement. So, we returned to the doctor's office for another prescription, and we were told to be patient.

A few days later, I noticed that Cameron was walking funny. He was not putting his right heel on the ground when he took a step. As I watched more closely, I saw that he couldn't straighten his right knee. It was swollen and he told me it hurt. Back to the pediatrician we went. This time, we were advised to try an over-the-counter NSAID.

As the weeks went by, the pain and swelling in Cameron's knee did not improve. Because I didn't want to wait to see our regular doctor, we took an appointment with a different pediatrician within the practice. After listening to our story and examining Cameron, she immediately suggested that we see a pediatric rheumatologist. I remember being surprised by that suggestion—what did she think it was? The doctor went on to explain that it could be a type of reactive arthritis (Cameron had strep throat just before school started), but she wanted to have him checked out. (Later, I found out this doctor also has psoriatic arthritis.)

When I called the department of rheumatology at our local children's hospital, I was speechless … they couldn't fit our son in until February or March, which was five months away! Because his knee was so swollen and painful, I told them I really didn't want to wait that long. Thankfully, they called another children's hospital about 90 miles away and got us an appointment two weeks later.

In the meantime, I remembered an online friend who has a child with arthritis. Even though we didn't have a diagnosis, I was anxious for more information. It was such a blessing to have someone to talk to who understood what our family was going through. Her child has psoriatic arthritis, and she was and still is very supportive!

At our first visit with the rheumatologist, Cameron was checked over thoroughly. It was brought to my attention that the ringworm we were treating was more than likely *not* ringworm, but psoriasis. She also noticed Cameron's nails. When he was about two years old, I had asked his pediatrician why his nails had so many pits in them and was told not to worry. As it turns out, he had the classic nail pitting found with psoriatic arthritis. Combined with the spot on his scalp, this led to a diagnosis of juvenile idiopathic arthritis (JIA)—psoriatic subtype. Psoriatic JIA is a disease of the immune system that causes raised red patches (psoriasis) on the skin, as well as pain, stiffness, and swelling of the joints. It can literally affect someone from head to toe. Left untreated, it can cause progressive joint damage. Cameron was also diagnosed with joint hypermobility syndrome, which means his joints can easily move beyond the normal range.

Our first step was to have Cameron's knee drained and injected with a steroid. When we arrived for his injection, the doctor noticed that his left knee had also started swelling, despite the fact that he had been taking naproxen for weeks. So, while he was under general anesthesia, she treated both knees.

At our follow-up appointment a month later, both of Cameron's knees were doing better. However, he had complained several times of some slight pain in his jaw while chewing. The doctor immediately scheduled him for an MRI, which revealed active arthritis on both sides of his jaw. We were shocked to find that he already had noticeable bone erosion! At that point, he started taking methotrexate along with a biologic drug to stop further damage to his joints.

He began his injections in late January 2010 and received his last injection in September 2012. Since then, he has been declared in remission. Cameron still has flares of psoriasis on his scalp and pain in his joints from time to time, but there is no active arthritis. While I'm thankful for his remission, I still hold my breath every time he complains of pain and each time we see the rheumatologist.

Recently, Cameron has been experiencing tachycardia (fast heart rate). When he goes from lying down to standing up, his heart rate shoots up, and he complains of a headache, dizziness, and what he calls "funky" vision. According to the rheumatologist, there is a documented link between hypermobility syndrome and postural orthostatic tachycardia syndrome (POTS). As a result, we are currently awaiting an evaluation with cardiology.

I find myself thinking about Cameron's future often. He will always need to be monitored for his arthritis and his psoriasis. I worry about whether his children will inherit this disease. I wonder if he will be able to do all the things he wants to do. Will his psoriasis get worse and affect other areas of his body? What are the long-term effects of the medications he has taken? These are just a few of the questions that swirl through my mind. But, thinking about these unknowns can make a person crazy, so I remind myself to take a step back and appreciate where he is today. Cameron is currently living without active arthritis. He is happy and doing well in school. And I have learned to live one day at a time.

Noah's Story by Caroline

When the oldest of our three boys was ten years old, he was a very active and talented baseball player. Noah had been playing baseball since he was four years old and had been selected to Little League All-Stars every season, as well as a travel team. He could play any position and, according to his coach, had the "best glove on the field." He was also the fastest runner, which is why it became concerning during his second season when he started complaining of being stiff in the mornings, having trouble running, and experiencing pain in his gluteal muscles (three muscles that comprise the buttocks).

Sometimes Noah would also complain that his lower back hurt, but mostly it was a vague pain and stiffness in his right gluteal. When he was catching for his team, we noticed he couldn't hop up from a squatting position and he looked very stiff. Mornings were the hardest.

We took him to his pediatrician who referred us to an orthopedist. They took X-rays of his pelvis and didn't see anything. Based on these results, as well as his examination, the doctor felt it was simply growing pains. This seemed plausible since, over the next year, Noah would have good days and bad days. Sometimes he felt great, hitting and pitching well, with no pain or stiffness. Other days he would say his shoulder hurt, he felt pain when he swung the bat, and his hip ached when he pitched.

Still concerned, we took him to a sports medicine doctor who X-rayed his shoulder but, again, found nothing. The doctor did say that he was surprised our son was a pitcher because his shoulder was so stiff. He recommended ibuprofen and rest. To loosen things up, the doctor showed Noah some exercises and stretches, which he performed daily. Noah loved baseball (and still does), so he was willing to do whatever was necessary to feel better. We even tried custom shoe inserts thinking it would help. But things did not improve.

In September, just two weeks after Noah started the sixth grade, we awoke to a scream in the middle of the night. When we raced into his room, our son said his back and hip were in such terrible pain that he couldn't move. I remember running my hands down his back and finding the area above his tailbone warm and swollen. And that's when I knew something was seriously wrong.

In the morning, we took Noah to a pediatric orthopedist in another city about an hour away. This time, when the doctor performed lab work he said the results were "alarming" and ordered an MRI to be done the same day. The results of the MRI were "nonspecific," meaning they saw something in his pelvis but they weren't sure what it was. We were referred to pediatric hematology at the children's hospital, where Noah was seen by an oncologist. Just the mention of cancer made this the scariest day of our lives. However, after more lab work and a thorough examination, the oncologist assured us she didn't think it was a malignancy.

We were then referred to pediatric rheumatology and had an appointment within days. Another MRI was ordered, this time with contrast, which revealed inflammation in Noah's pelvis; a rather rare finding for a child of twelve. More specifically, our son was diagnosed with HLA-B27 juvenile spondyloarthropathy associated ankylosing spondylitis, a type of juvenile arthritis. We finally had a diagnosis, and although we were relieved there were no malignancies, we faced a different set of worries.

As a mother and a registered nurse, I experienced a lot of guilt after Noah's diagnosis. I felt I should have known; I should have understood how much he was hurting and kept taking him to the doctor. However, because his pain and stiffness seemed to come and go, growing pains seemed like a logical explanation. What I've since learned about this disease is that it goes in and out of remission. Stress can trigger a "flare up" and sometimes it just happens. When these flares occur, our pediatric rheumatologist only has a handful of "tricks she can pull out of her black bag," because, unfortunately, there are not a lot of treatment options available. There is also currently no cure.

It's been five years since Noah was diagnosed, and I'm happy to say he's doing great. His inflammation is controlled with medication, and he has a great attitude. He is currently attending early college/high school and hopes to study for a career in the healthcare field where he can help children with inflammatory arthritis.

While the exact cause of JA is unknown, scientists believe genetics play a role. The genetic marker HLA-B27 is often found in those with juvenile spondyloarthropathy. Our youngest son, who is nine years old, has tested positive for this marker and is currently being evaluated by Noah's pediatric rheumatologist. He is exhibiting some signs of inflammation and occasionally complains of gluteal and ankle pain, but is not on any medication at this time. Thankfully, our middle son does not appear to have any signs or symptoms of inflammatory arthritis. It remains a genetic mystery, however, since nobody in our family has had this disease. Though neither I nor my husband has JA, one of us must be positive for the gene—what triggers it is unknown.

Going forward, we are optimistic that research will provide additional treatment options, and that more medical professionals will choose pediatric rheumatology as a specialty (like our son!). More importantly, we remain hopeful that a cure will be found.

Solving Allie's Mystery by Allie

My name is Allie, and for three years I was a medical mystery. It all began when I was 13 years old and went to the pediatrician for a regular checkup. My mom mentioned to the doctor that I looked "swollen" and had frequent back pain. At first we thought hormones may be causing the swelling and that my heavy backpack was the culprit behind the back pain. But the swelling was constant, not just once a month, and lightening the load in my backpack really didn't help with the back pain. The doctor ordered some blood work to see what might be going on. When the results came back, he called my mom and asked to see her in his office, which meant the news wasn't good. The blood work indicated poor kidney function, and we were referred to nephrology—a branch of medicine that deals with kidneys.

The nephrologist conducted more tests, including an antinuclear antibody (ANA) analysis, a blood test used to screen for autoimmune disorders. The test came up negative, but the doctor explained that just because it was negative at the time didn't mean it wouldn't test positive later. Based on my symptoms, he suspected I had systemic lupus erythematosus (SLE), commonly called lupus, which is a chronic autoimmune disease that may affect the skin, joints, kidneys, brain, and other organs. Like other autoimmune disorders, the body's immune system mistakenly attacks healthy issue, which leads to inflammation, pain, and possible damage to the areas being attacked. Symptoms vary from person-to-person and may come and go (flares and remissions). The doctor said my case was very similar to some of the other young patients he had in his clinic, but it was too early to make a definitive diagnosis. Therefore, I was listed with "nonspecific autoimmune disease."

My nephrologist was an amazing doctor because he really listened to us. Unfortunately, we had to move and I started seeing new doctors in rheumatology. By this time I was nearly 15 years old, and though I was still having symptoms, no one had given us a firm diagnosis. At my first appointment with these new doctors, I was discouraged because I felt they weren't really listening. In fact, they tried to explain away all my symptoms, telling my mom there was nothing wrong with me except taking in too many calories—which was not true! I barely ate lunch at school and was careful to eat healthy meals at home. Needless to say, we were very frustrated—all we wanted was an accurate diagnosis so I could be properly treated. We went to many other doctors looking for an answer, and along the way I was suspected of having fibromyalgia, lymphedema, lupus, and a few other autoimmune disorders.

Finally, a month after my sixteenth birthday, I had my first appointment at the University of Florida Academic Health Center (Shands) and met my current rheumatologist. He listened to my story, reviewed my very thick medical file, asked a lot of questions, and performed a thorough examination. When he was done, he diagnosed me with lupus nephritis (inflammation of the kidneys) and juvenile arthritis, which are closely related. I learned that many lupus sufferers also develop lupus nephritis (up to 60 percent according to the National Institutes of Health) and frequently develop arthritis.

Though it was scary to hear, putting a name to my "nonspecific autoimmune disease" was a relief, because not knowing what I had for three years and looking for an answer were very stressful. I felt like a complicated puzzle with a missing piece or a mystery that couldn't be solved. Finding a solution meant that I could finally get proper treatment. I am now on daily medication and receive a chemo infusion every three months to help control my lupus and maintain normal kidney function. It's not easy, but it's a great feeling knowing that I'm getting the treatment I need—and to no longer be a mystery.

CHAPTER FOUR

The Team Approach

Now that you've learned a little about the opponent and met a few players, it's time for you to assemble your own team ... your healthcare team, that is. Treatment plans for juvenile arthritis (JA) are highly individualized because each child responds differently to medications and therapies and may have varied body parts and systems that are affected. This is why it's so important to select the right healthcare team for *your* child. Both my children have JIA, but their medical teams have a different lineup. Evan has a rheumatologist, ophthalmologist, orthopedist, and immunologist. Grant's list of specialists is more extensive, but it no longer includes a doctor of immunology. Because their cases and manifestations are so diverse, they each need a unique set of professionals to provide the proper care.

Building Your Roster

Leading this team of specialists is the rheumatologist, since JA is at the root of the related health issues your child may face. Once a diagnosis is obtained, he or she can begin steering you in the right direction; helping you to decide whether you need another specialist or just a follow-up visit with your pediatrician or rheumatologist. In most cases, your roster of specialists will include an ophthalmologist.

Children with any form of autoimmune disease will typically be referred to an ophthalmologist, as they run a higher risk of developing inflammatory conditions in the eyes—some with very serious ramifications if not caught early enough. The most common eye issue is *uveitis* or inflammation of the inner eye. You may also hear the term *iritis* mentioned, which refers to a specific form of uveitis that affects the iris. Although some eye issues are caused by JA, others may be triggered by the medications used to treat it. These conditions usually develop slowly, so early intervention is key to the prevention of permanent damage. As a result, regular and sometimes more frequent visits to the ophthalmologist are recommended for children with rheumatic diseases.

A PERFECT FIT FOR JENNA by AMY

Some parents remember every detail of their child's diagnosis, but for me those first weeks are a blur of events and emotions. What really stands out in my mind was how small and vulnerable my daughter was and how helpless I felt. It was the summer of 2008, and Jenna, the youngest of my three children, was just 4½ years old. After my husband and my mother both commented on the size and shape of her knees on the same day, I knew something must be wrong. The very next day we took her in to see our family physician. Unlike many families who have to wait months for a diagnosis, our doctor immediately suspected juvenile arthritis. At the time, we were living in Maine, which does not have a pediatric rheumatologist, so our doctor referred us to one of only a few adult rheumatologists who are willing to see children.

Jenna's first appointment with the rheumatologist revealed more inflamed joints, in addition to the fluid on both knees. Further tests confirmed the diagnosis of juvenile arthritis. I suppose I should have been shocked to hear that, but I wasn't—at least not yet. I remember thinking, "Okay, she will take some medication and be okay." But, of course, this disease is more complicated than that.

Based on her lab work, the rheumatologist told us that Jenna needed to be seen by an eye doctor immediately. At this point, I thought he was crazy—arthritis in her eyes? I continued to question this when I called to schedule an appointment with our regular eye doctor, but they confirmed that arthritis can indeed affect the eyes and is a very serious condition. In fact, they fit us in the next day.

At her first appointment, we were told that Jenna's eyes were fine, but the doctor wanted to see her weekly. She reiterated that uveitis, which is basically inflammation of the eye, is a dangerous, silent, quick-moving condition. I took her words to heart, and although the eye doctor was about an hour drive each way, we agreed to weekly appointments. It was on our third visit that the doctor discovered uveitis. I could tell that she felt heartsick for us.

We were sent home with three bottles of eye drops, but our optometrist could no longer help us with this condition. It was time to see an oph-thalmologist. Again, Maine had only one pediatric ophthalmologist at the time, and, unfortunately, he was not a good fit for us. After leaving an appointment with both Jenna and I in tears, I vowed to find a different doctor. By this time, the inflammation was increasing due to the uveitis, and the pressures in her eyes were building due to the steroid eye drops. To make matters worse, the arthritis in her joints was not being properly controlled.

During these very difficult days, we learned two lessons: (1) an adult rheumatologist does not always know how to treat a pediatric case, and (2) just because it's a pediatric office does not mean the doctor has any business treating children. For a period of time we were driving three hours each way to see a different doctor in Cambridge for Jenna's uveitis. The drive was tedious, but this doctor was a perfect fit! However, Jenna's adult rheumatologist was not willing to change her course of treatment and work with the ophthalmologist.

Initially, I felt powerless—I am not a doctor, I thought, I'm just a parent. What can I do? Then one day our rheumatologist mentioned that he knew one of the residents at Duke Children's Hospital. He asked if we had considered the possibility of moving. Because we were so frustrated with watching our daughter deteriorate, at the age of four, we were willing to consider anything. So, a plan was set into motion.

In June 2009, we moved from Maine to North Carolina to get Jenna the medical care she so desperately needed, as well as to get her into a warmer climate. It was early fall before we were able to get an appointment with the pediatric rheumatologists and ophthalmologists at Duke. We had still been administering eye drops several times a day, and Jenna was taking NSAIDs and methotrexate daily, as well as a biologic drug every other week. During her first appointment at Duke, all the doctors agreed that the mix of drugs had to change; they weren't doing anything for the uveitis. Since our previous medical team had disagreed about medications, it was refreshing to have all the doctors on the same page!

Within three months of her new treatment, both Jenna's eyes and joints were *all clear*! Talk about relief! From December 2009 to January

2013, Jenna experienced periodic, minor flare ups of her arthritis, which meant she had to stay on her meds, but her eyes have not flared at all. In January 2013, we began the process of weaning Jenna off of her medications. I was told this could take up to a year to do successfully, during which her doctors will monitor her closely. But, for now, she is on her way to a full remission!

If I could stress only one thing to other parents who are dealing with this disease, it would be—do your own research. Don't assume the doctor treating your child has been trained properly on this condition. With so few uveitis specialists, let alone pediatric uveitis specialists, it can be difficult to get proper treatment. It took us many months to find the right team of medical specialists (and a move to a new state), but seeing my daughter on the road to remission is worth every effort.

An ophthalmologist, along with your rheumatologist and pediatrician, will be the core group of your medical team, while other specialists will vary based on the type of JA your child has, as well as the manifestations of the disease they suffer with the most. Early in Grant's case, the most prevalent JA-related issues fell under the dermatology and gastroenterology departments, but in Evan's case, immunology played a more important role. Since a large percentage of lupus patients suffer from nephritis (inflammation of the kidneys), a nephrologist is often consulted, while in other forms of JA it may never be an issue.

As the disease evolves, your team may also need to change. For example, in the last year or so, Grant's gastrointestinal issues have become almost nonexistent, and he has been able to spread his follow-up appointments out to yearly visits (unless of course something else changes). The rashes that plagued him and were being followed by dermatology are now so mild or infrequent that they can be managed through his rheumatologist and pediatrician. Although we have been able to let a few of our specialists go, which is a wonderful thing (from both sides!), we have picked up a few others along the way. As our situation has changed, so has Grant's "dream team." Currently, endocrinology is playing a key role in his treatment plan, but in time that may change as well.

Managing the Team

For parents, working with multiple doctors can be overwhelming. A full schedule of hospital, doctor, and clinic visits can be taxing for your child as well. It's difficult to be poked, prodded, and asked the same questions multiple times in the same week, or even the same day! With that in mind, although it's often necessary to see a long list of specialists, we try to streamline the team whenever possible. With the guidance of our current doctors, we periodically choose which areas are the most critical, and in which areas we can focus less, or perhaps have another doctor pull double duty.

There is also something to be said for "too many cooks in the kitchen." While it's important to keep regular appointments with the specialists your child needs, a complicated case can make communication between multiple doctors more challenging—and the potential for mistakes can increase. One area where this is likely to happen is with medications. Although doctors do their best to check for drug-to-drug interactions, many pharmaceuticals are not commonly known or used across different disciplines. With thousands of drugs on the market, all with warnings and indications that constantly change (not to mention the possibility of parent error in reporting a current medication from one doctor to the next), counter-indication accidents can occur. At times, Grant's list of medications was so long and changed so frequently that even I made occasional mistakes in reporting what he was taking from one visit to the next—and I was the one giving all the medications!

That's why the pharmacist should be considered a very important part of your child's medical team. The more complicated your child's case may become, the more critical it will be to have *one* person who follows every drug prescribed and can be on the lookout for potential issues. More than once our pharmacist has found possible drug-to-drug interactions and was able to contact the doctors and find a safer alternative. On at least one occasion, our pharmacist discovered that a prescribed drug converted into sulfa in the body (although it was not a sulfa drug, per se) and could trigger another severe allergic reaction, based on Grant's history!

Most pharmacists can also provide you with a printout of all the medications your child is taking, along with the dosages. I always ask the doctor to update a prescription dosage change with the pharmacy as it happens, which is a simple process with today's technology. Taking a copy of this up-to-date record of all medications to each doctor's visit helps reduce potential errors and is another way to ensure your child is getting the best possible treatment.

Looking at the Big Picture

Even after you've assembled a team of top-notch specialists in every area of concern and enlisted the help of a great pharmacist who can assist you in medication safety and administration, you are left with the most important job: managing the care of the *whole* child. As specialists focus on their individual areas of know-how, the big picture can sometimes be overlooked. Your child is not merely a sum of parts, but a unique individual with a complex condition. So, while all those specialists may be "right" regarding their point of expertise, they can also be missing something important.

Have you ever heard the story of the blind men and the elephant? Many Asian cultures have their own spin on this parable, but the essence of the story goes like this: Several blind men were led to an elephant and asked to describe what they "saw." The first said, "This creature is much like a tree—broad, circular, and standing strong!" Another responded that the first man was all wrong; the creature was thin and large, like a paper fan, moving the air and creating a breeze. The third man scoffed at the other two, smugly noting that the animal in question was small and resembled a paintbrush, while another described what he observed as a hose to transport water. The last man stated that all the others were wrong: It was a massive creature, built large and solid, like a house! All were firm in their observations and argued who was right.

In fact, they were all correct. The first man had been led to the elephant's leg, the second to its ear, the third to its tail (with a tuft of hair at the end), the fourth to its trunk, and the last to the body. Although each one of them accurately described a part of the elephant, none of them had captured the essence of the *whole* animal. Specialists specialize! In many ways, they can be like the blind men in this story, focusing so hard on one aspect (which is their job) that the overall picture of your child's health can be skewed by their expertise. That's where the pediatrician comes in.

Arguably, I would say the pediatrician could be *the* most important member of your child's team. As generalists, they are trained to see the big picture. Additionally, your pediatrician will probably have known your child longer than any of the other specialists. He or she has the advantage of history and a personal relationship with your child—kind of like a third parent with a medical degree.

The pediatrician is your first line of defense against this disease and the bridge between your family and the entire team of specialists. Your pediatrician, in addition to providing routine care, can serve as a point person to coordinate the medical team, making sure the big picture isn't overlooked and keeping everyone connected. If the pediatrician observes what you've been seeing and conveys it to the rest of the team, there is instantly more credibility and a faster call to action.

Access to your pediatric rheumatologist may be difficult, so utilizing your pediatrician first, and the rheumatologist later, is a solid plan of action. Consider that in the United States, there are approximately 300,000 children with some type of juvenile arthritis—and only about 200 pediatric rheumatologists in the entire country. In fact, at least eight states do not even *have* a pediatric rheumatologist! Worldwide, this shortage of pediatric rheumatologists is even more acute, with estimates coming in at a total of 250! In some cases, adult rheumatologists must follow pediatric cases due to a lack of resources; and since pediatric cases differ greatly from adult onset arthritis, the pediatrician's input becomes even more critical.

Finding the Right Fit

With the pediatrician playing such an important role in your child's care, it's very important to find a doctor who is "right" for both you and your child. Early in Grant's diagnosis, we changed pediatricians. Although we really liked our pediatrician and had no complaints, our rheumatologist recommended another doctor with a little more experience in complicated autoimmune cases—a doctor with whom *she* already had a good rapport. We interviewed the new pediatrician and liked him a lot, so we decided to make the switch to strengthen the team.

It's not always that easy. In some cases, you may find that a doctor is knowledgeable but has no bedside manner, or that he/she doesn't mesh well with your child. You are going to be seeing a lot of these folks, and, in general, the experience is already trying. If your child has a strong dislike for the doctor, and there are other good options available, then spare yourself the grief and find someone they like and trust. The same holds true if *you* don't have faith in the doctor. Even if a doctor is well respected and gets along with your child, if you find yourself always second guessing his or her opinions or have difficulty communicating and resolving issues, it may be time to find another physician. It's hard enough managing the care of a chronically ill child; if at all possible, you shouldn't have to bear the burden of dealing with a difficult team member.

Unfortunately, you may not always have a choice. Your insurance might dictate whom you can see, or the distance you have to travel to see a rheumatologist may be the deciding factor. Friends of ours who have a child with juvenile myositis (JM) have been forced to change rheumatologists three times—once for insurance reasons, once due to the doctor's retirement, and another because the doctor was leaving their medical group. It can be extremely frustrating to have to start over with a new doctor, but in all three instances, this family made the best of the situation and kept a positive attitude, which is important.

Your child is always looking up to you, including the way you handle the challenges and deal with the circumstances surrounding their medical condition. If they see that you have questions and concerns about the quality of care they are receiving, it only heightens their anxiety. You will have to work that much harder to advocate for your child behind the scenes, educate yourself, and build a better relationship with each new doctor. Again, these are the times that a wonderful pediatrician is invaluable as a respected, knowledgeable supporter and a necessary go-between who can provide continuity in their care.

Communicating Effectively

Who knows your child best? Who has the biggest stake in their health? Who loves and cares about them the most? You as the parents do. While the doctors are concerned about your child's health, they have many patients and limited time (especially the rheumatologists!). It's tempting as a parent, who desperately wants to make their kids "all better," to provide the doctor with as much information as possible. Big mistake.

You can positively affect your child's care by learning how to communicate effectively with the doctor. It's a delicate balance between providing thorough information and overwhelming the doctor with ancillary facts. Your time with the doctor will always be limited, and even during rough patches, such as a flare, they may not be able to see your child right away. Remember, there are 300,000 kids and only about 200 doctors trained to treat them. So, what can you do to make the most of your time with your child's doctor? Plenty!

Keep a Journal

Start the journal and do it religiously. After all, now that you've educated yourself and you know what to look for, as well as how to

TIPS FOR MAKING THE MOST OF YOUR DOCTOR'S VISITS

Be Prepared
- Write down any questions you have and bring them with you.
- Bring your journal or other notes, along with photos.
- If it's a new doctor or there have been recent changes, be sure to bring an up-to-date list of medications/dosages.

Be Brief
- Stick to the facts.
- Answer questions as succinctly as possible.
- Talk to the staff about non-doctor issues such as prescriptions and school notes.

Take Notes

Don't Get Emotional

recognize subtle changes in your child, you can record pertinent information. While helpful to the doctor, this journal is really for you. Write down *everything* you think could be relevant. For instance, if your child develops a rash, record what type of rash it was, when it began, and how long it stayed, along with what helped or didn't help. Was there a fever? If so, how high did it get and how long did it persist? Did your child experience joint pain? Where was it and were the joints swollen, hot, and red or all of the above? Was there a "bug" going around school that they could have picked up? Are there any other strange symptoms, such as difficulty sleeping after a new medication was prescribed or unusual fatigue? Don't forget to include the date along with the details. I kept a page in a spiral notebook for each day, even if I wrote "pretty good day" because there were no big issues.

While it may seem like just one more thing to do, this journal will help you identify patterns that you can summarize for the doctor. For example, when Grant was taking methotrexate, I noticed that he was overly nauseated and developed a lot of headaches—even compared to what other parents had told me their children were experiencing on the same medication. I noted the pattern: Exactly four hours after taking the drug, he would wake up in the middle of the night vomiting and be out of commission for the next 24–48 hours. Armed with this specific information regarding timing, the doctor suggested a dissolvable anti-nausea pill that I could give my son in the middle of the night without waking him. That took care of the nausea, and the extra sleep alleviated the headaches. The outcome may have been very different if I had vaguely described how the medication made him sick all the time. With this information, observed over time, I was able to give the doctor just what was needed to solve the problem.

Take Pictures

In the beginning, Grant also developed a lot of strange, inconsistent rashes. Many times, I would try to describe a rash to the doctor (or the phone nurse), who would invariably suggest that I bring him into the office. However, by the time we got there, the rash would be gone! As you can imagine, this was very frustrating for all parties. The solution was just a "click away." I began taking photos of the rashes as they occurred.

Keeping a photographic journal also worked well when Evan started to show signs of swollen joints. I took photos, in good light, until I had captured the way the swelling looked in real life. Then I took more, noting the times, so that when I did visit the doctor, he could see how the cycles evolved and over what time frame. Since Evan was negative for inflammatory markers on his initial labs, this photographic evidence was the first thing to alert the doctors that he may actually have JIA. The photos, coupled with a visit during which he started to show signs of the same cycle, helped the doctor make his diagnosis.

Photographs serve as an objective observation tool for doctors when they cannot be present. While it's certainly more fun to catalog photos of sporting events or special occasions, I have found it very helpful to sort these medical photos into organized files (i.e., skin rashes, joints, and eyes). As a result, I can tell the doctor that Grant developed a strange rash in conjunction with a flare, or that we saw a different type of rash cycle around the time a medication was administered, or whatever the case may be. The photos, together with my notes regarding timing and other symptoms, provide the doctor with a very clear, unbiased picture of what is happening when they are unable to observe it firsthand.

Be Brief

Another great tip when communicating with doctors is to try to be brief. Give the facts and stick to them. Answer their questions as succinctly as possible. If some issues can be addressed with the nurse (such as e-prescribing to a different pharmacy or putting in a request for a note for school, etc.), then do that instead. Save the issues that only the doctor can address for the doctor, and let the other things be handled by the staff whenever possible. It's also helpful to ask your pediatrician for his or her opinion before calling the rheumatologist. Grant's pediatrician prefers e-mail. If I have a pressing question, I will e-mail him with the situation and ask if we can we take care of it without a trip to the rheumatologist. Many times, the pediatrician is able to help with the problem or, if necessary, get a faster response from the specialist.

Leave Emotions at Home

Try to keep emotion out of it—I know that's tough advice to follow, but I have learned over the years that emotional visits can take a toll on the doctors, as well as you, while making your appointments less productive. By staying calm and professional and providing the necessary information, you're helping the doctor to do a better job. Give the physician a chance to address your concerns, and though it may seem like an obvious and simple courtesy, remember to say "thank you." Like any other ongoing relationship, it should be treated with respect.

There is nothing wrong with being emotional about this disease and expressing your feelings about the things your child, your family, and you are going through. However, the clinic visit is not the time to address it. Have your questions ready and written down so you don't forget, and hold the emotion for a counselor, if necessary. Getting weepy over bad news during the visit will only make it more difficult to find out everything you need to know while you have the doctor in the room with you. And perhaps, most importantly, it will upset your child. Be strong then, and find your release elsewhere.

The Insurance Company

The medical team is not the only group with whom you will need to communicate effectively. Although it sometimes *feels* like an adversarial partnership, your insurance company is a very important factor in securing the right treatment for your child. Be nice, but push when necessary. Our insurance processors know me by name! There are also tips and tricks you can use to get the most mileage out of your insurance coverage and facilitate the process (see sidebar). The sooner you learn the ins and outs of your insurance company and your particular policy, the easier the process becomes. Like everything else, there is a learning curve, but once you begin to understand the way things work, you can handle the procedures with less frustration and more efficiency.

NEVER TAKE "No" FOR AN ANSWER! by MONICA

(Tips for Working with Your Insurance Company)

Having an ill child is tough enough. The last thing you need is what can seem like a nonstop battle with the insurance companies. Allow me to help. As a mother, medical professional, and former insurance company employee, I have the unique perspective of seeing this situation from all sides. I have been a registered nurse for more than 20 years. Nearly 13 years ago I became the mother of a wonderful child. Due to his health problems, I took a job working for a major health insurance company. During that time, I picked up some tips that every parent of a chronically ill child (or anyone else who has dealt with an insurance company) should know.

The first step is to read your medical policy. It sounds like common sense, but much like the manual that comes with a new appliance, very few people take the time to actually read it. When dealing with major health issues, it's important to be *very* familiar with your policy—paying close attention to areas regarding "pre-certification" or "pre-notification." Often, the insurance company must be contacted *prior* to surgeries or diagnostic imaging (such as MRI or CT scans). Even if no further information is required, a call must be placed in order for the benefits to be paid. This may also be the case with hospital admissions and visits to the emergency room. When in doubt, call the pre-certification number on your card. If you are told that pre-certification is not needed, ask for the name of the person with whom you are speaking and record the date and time you called. Better to be safe than to receive a surprise bill as a result of not following "the rules."

The same process applies to pharmacy claims, which are often managed by a different company than your major medical coverage. At times, your pharmacy vendor will indicate that a medication should be covered by major medical, while major medical will indicate that pharmacy should cover it. (This is often the case with expensive "specialty tier" medications.) Reading through both policies may help to clarify. If it doesn't, ask to set up a conference call with a representative from each side to resolve the issue. Again, it's important to get the names of the people with whom you speak and record the time and date of the call. If the representative references a medical policy, rule, or a specific exclusion, ask them to e-mail or fax a copy to you for review, and keep it for your records.

Sometimes a service that is not normally covered by your policy, such as eye exams, may be covered under major medical due to its classification. With JA, eye exams can often be covered as part of the prevention and treatment of inflammation due to disease, rather than under the umbrella of vision benefits, which may not be covered at all.

This brings us to the most hated part of dealing with an insurance company: *Denials!* When you receive the denial of a claim or a pre-certification, don't panic. Denials don't always mean no. In fact, a very large number of claims are simply denied for something termed "Lack of Medical Information." This is as simple as it sounds; the claim or pre-certification was submitted either with no supporting medical information or did not contain the necessary information to garner approval. The letter you receive should detail the information needed to complete the review, which will likely be approved the second time around.

You may be wondering "why don't insurance companies tell people up front what they want to know?" This up-front information is especially important for things such as growth hormones, injections, orthotics, wheelchairs, and other high-cost items. Actually, insurance companies *do* let you know what information is needed. They are required by law to publish all medical policies on their websites. The trick is in finding them. In most cases, you can locate the company's main website and then look for the "Provider" area. Once there, search for a section that refers to "Standards" and then find "Medical Policy." At this point, many sites will ask you to agree to their terms of use before proceeding—just say "yes." Now you can look for the specific procedure, test, or surgery. The exact information required will be spelled out. Print this page and take it to your physician if you are being referred to a specialist for something specific. Forwarding this information will help prevent the denial in the first place. It can also avert the need for a second visit to your physician (and second co-pay) to test something they didn't realize the insurance company required.

If the claim is truly denied based on medical reasons, ask for an appeal and request a review by an independent third party. For off-label use of medications or treatments, determine their exception rules and ask your provider to submit the necessary information. Sometimes it can be as simple as the provider submitting several peer-published journal articles supporting the off-label use. It's all about getting the right information in the right hands, at the right time.

And now for those pesky documents known as Explanations of Benefits (EOBs). If you're like most people, you don't bother to read through the EOBs you receive. But it's important to match your medical bills to those EOBs for several reasons. The first is to be sure your provider remembers to take off any insurance discounts. The amount allowed is *rarely* what is billed, and if you are in-network for most PPOs or HMOs, the provider is to discount anything above the allowed/negotiated amount. Occasionally providers send a bill after the insurance company issues the EOB, and the discount is not removed until you call. When in doubt, call the billing office at your provider and ask them to explain why you are being asked to pay what appeared to be the network discount.

The second reason to review the EOB is for tax purposes. Talk to a tax professional or review the IRS website to determine what is considered a medical expense. If you meet the guidelines or think it might be close, keep *everything*, including those EOBs.

Reviewing your EOBs can also help prevent a rising and costly problem—the theft of health insurance benefits/insurance fraud. Review each EOB to be sure you saw the provider on the indicated day and that all services billed appear to be what was provided for the right family member. I once reviewed a file where a child's entire cancer treatment was billed under both the child and the mother (double billed), due to what the provider reported was a system error. In another instance, the cancer treatment being billed was done in California, but the insured patient lived in Illinois. Insurance companies are working to stop this type of fraud, but it's very important to watch for it yourself. If you notice any irregularities, contact both the insurance company and the provider billing office.

I realize this may seem like a lot to take on, especially when you're caring for a sick child. Trust me, I've been there. It can, at times, seem like a full-time job. If possible, consider delegating whatever you can to a family member or friend who has asked what they can do to help. The insurance company may not talk to them for you, but they can do the research. Also, some insurance companies will allow you to designate a person to communicate with them. Don't be afraid to ask.

Finally, ask your insurance company or the hospital where your child's specialists practice if they have case managers assigned to assist patients/families with medical care. These people are not only experienced with the ins and outs of insurance issues, they can also help arrange outpatient services such as physical, occupational, or speech therapy. In addition, there is a growing business of professionals called healthcare advocates, who can help you navigate insurance companies, pharmacies, hospitals, and more. While there are many great ones out there, beware of scammers; be sure to research the organization fully prior to signing a contract. Insurance does not cover the services of these advocates, but the time and aggravation from which they can save you could be well worth the cost.

A few more helpful hints:

- If the paperwork seems overwhelming, try to tackle a little at a time.
- If your insurance company offers "e-mail us," use it. Communicating in this way leaves a helpful paper trail and can be accessed night or day.
- If you prefer to communicate by phone, be sure to take good notes.
- When dealing with a problem, try to remember that it isn't personal, even when it feels that way.
- When it seems like all the insurance company says is "No," remember that the person on the other end of the line hates the word *no* just as much as you do. Yelling will not help! The person you are talking to does not get a bonus for denying your claim. In fact, most companies have to submit regular reports to the government to prove they aren't denying things incorrectly. All denials must also be signed off by at least one physician.
- Please be kind to the reps. They are following very tight rules that are actually set forth and enforced by the government to make sure everyone is treated fairly.

Cutting Costs

Even with insurance coverage, treatments and medications can still be expensive. The good news is there are some options that can help you manage these additional costs, regardless of your family income. If you haven't dealt with a chronic illness before, you may not be aware of the programs that are out there or some of the steps you can take to decrease the financial burden.

Begin by talking to the hospital or billing office. I was shocked when I called the hospital to correct a billing error and was offered an additional discount after the correction was made. Since we had a large bill, and I was discussing (civilly, I might add) the remaining costs with the representative, she told me she was authorized to extend me an additional courtesy discount. I paid the balance that day, but with a significant savings, even from the adjusted bill. Had I not called to discuss the error, I would have never known that negotiating with the hospital was even an option! I asked some other parents in my chronically ill child community about this phenomenon and found others had the same experience. It may not happen every time, but it never hurts to ask.

Another place you can discover savings is with the pharmaceutical companies. With a little research, you can find many ways to spread your dollar further. Most do not advertise coupons or co-pay assist programs, but many of them have options, especially for expensive medications (see "Maximize Your Medication Dollars" for more tips).

From your trusted pediatrician and the many specialists you may see, to the local pharmacist and your insurance company, all play an important role on your child's medical team. By communicating effectively with these professionals and taking the time to develop strong relationships, you can help to ensure that your child receives the best care possible—and a difficult process can be a little less stressful.

MAXIMIZE YOUR MEDICATION DOLLARS by MONICA

Medication can be expensive, especially when it comes to the specialty drugs often prescribed for JA. But there are ways to maximize your medication dollars.

- If your child is taking a name-brand medication, visit the company's website and look for coupons that can be used toward the co-pay. Some of these coupons will reduce a $100.00 co-pay to $10.00, while others offer the first 30 days free! This is particularly helpful if your child has allergies or issues tolerating medications. There is nothing more frustrating than paying a $65.00 co-pay, only to have your child break out in a head-to-toe rash after two days.

- Don't be afraid to ask your physician if there is a generic alternative. Unfortunately, for many of the "orphan diseases" there are no good generics. If that's the case, ask your physician to work with the representatives to provide samples.

- If you are on a limited budget, check the drug manufacturer's website to determine if they have an assistance program. Don't assume you earn too much money. If there is nothing offered on their website, find a "contact us" and e-mail them. Explain your story. Even if it results in a voucher for a one month's supply, your efforts will have paid off.

- Consider the pharmacy you use to fill prescriptions. Many of the major discount stores (Walmart, Meijer, Kmart) have much lower costs on generics than your standard co-pay. At the time of this writing, Meijer offered many free generic antibiotics.

- Check out the Partnership for Prescription Assistance www.pparx.org, which offers a one-stop place to check for assistance programs.

THE PEDIATRICIAN'S WISH LIST by DR. JOSHUA LEVIN

In order to get the most out of your visit with the pediatrician, it's critical that he or she has all of the necessary information to best help your child. While this may sound simple, juvenile arthritis patients often have complicated cases, involving a large amount of information to track. Therefore, it's important to be organized, both mentally and with your notes, so you can accurately answer your pediatrician's questions, and he or she can answer yours. Effectively communicating the details of your child's care is the key to a productive visit: It will enable the team approach to thrive and provide top-notch medical care for your family.

Your appointment actually starts well before you arrive at the pediatrician's office by being fully prepared and organized. You can compile information in many different ways, including spiral notebooks, laptops, or iPads. It doesn't matter which method you choose, as long as the information is well organized and easily accessible. Keeping a journal is a great way to track your child's symptoms and reveal possible patterns. Your journal should include vital signs, such as your child's temperature, as well as medications you administered and whether or not they worked, foods your child has eaten, sleep patterns, new illnesses, and any other symptoms or changes you observe.

For physicians, especially those who treat rheumatologic issues, identifying patterns is critical to solving problems. For example, one form of arthritis can flare after eating gluten, which makes tracking dietary habits important. In addition to written notes, taking photos is an excellent way to document rashes and other medical findings such as red eyes, swollen joints, or mouth sores. As they say, a picture can speak a thousand words—conveying valuable information that may be difficult to relay with simple explanations. Bringing your notes or journal with you to the pediatrician's office will not only help you relay information to the physician, but also allow you to take goods notes during the appointment. Chances are you will want to refer back to these notes, either at home while caring for your child or at a visit with another member of the medical team. It will further enhance the team's ability to function together as a unit to care for your child.

To start the visit, the pediatrician needs to know *exactly* why you are there. In medicine, we call it the "chief complaint." In other words, what is your primary goal for the visit? By being clear on what needs to be accomplished, you can help guide your pediatrician in the direction he or she needs to go with this appointment. Is your child running a fever, or is there a new rash? Do you need refills on certain medications, but are unsure if the dose is correct? Are you having trouble reaching your specialist and want the pediatrician to help bridge the communication gap? All of these are common reasons for seeing the pediatrician, and being clear on your objectives is step one of a productive visit. Whatever the issues may be, be sure to clearly and concisely communicate your specific goals at the outset.

As the visit progresses, focus on communicating well and working as a team. Be sure to have the latest, most updated medical information to give to the pediatrician. A current list of medications, including dosages and when they are administered, is vital. These medications may change regularly, and being current will help address how well they are working, what side effects might be occurring, and what changes may be needed. It can also be helpful to have a copy of the notes or letters from recent visits with the specialist, so the pediatrician can be up to speed on the latest recommendations. At a minimum, bring your own notes from the specialist visit, so if information has not been received by the pediatrician, you can fill in the gaps. In some cases, the specialist may send a letter to your pediatrician by fax or mail, but this is not always the case. Therefore, if you provide a synopsis of the specialist visit, you can be certain that your pediatrician and specialist will be on the same page.

At the conclusion of the visit, review in your own mind the goals you had. Have your concerns been addressed? Do you fully understand the plan put forth to care for your child? It can be frustrating to arrive home and realize you forgot to ask an important question, or that you don't really understand the physician's directions. Be sure to ask questions about any lingering issues, but be respectful of the pediatrician's time. It's important to have reasonable expectations for each visit, which is why it's so valuable to have your list of goals thought out ahead of time. By reviewing them again at the end of the visit, you can be sure you've achieved your objectives, which is what both you and your pediatrician want.

Finally, if there are any items your pediatrician has asked you to follow-up on, be certain to do so. Follow-up and an ongoing line of communication with your pediatrician are critical. This will allow the physician to maintain an overview of your child's care and remain up-to-date on progress made since the office visit. Different pediatricians will vary in their preferred method of communication, so be sure to discuss that and confirm how best to follow-up. With regular follow-up and thorough, updated communication, your pediatrician will be able to effectively serve as the quarterback of your child's medical team.

CHAPTER FIVE

The Head Coach

Every team needs a great head coach. In 1999, my husband was playing pro football for the St. Louis Rams. The year before, his team was tied with another franchise for the "most losing team of the decade." Not a great title to have! Although the talent base on the team was very similar to the season before, the head coach Dick Vermeil had just enough time to whip his team into shape, utilize his leadership skills, and take that losing team all the way to the Super Bowl—with a third string quarterback, no less!

That was a magic season. We had all been feeling the effects of so many losing seasons prior to that year, and having both our starting quarterback and his backup out felt like insurmountable obstacles … but not to Coach. He knew the team intimately and put everyone in the right place at the right time. He motivated with his leadership and his true concern for every player. We were the longest shot for the Super Bowl, but we won it all. And the talent he recognized in that third string quarterback? Well, football fans may remember him better by name—Kurt Warner.

In the same way that Coach Vermeil was such an instrumental part of the Ram's success, *you* play a huge role in the success your family will have in fighting this disease. You are the head coach in your child's battle against JA. Even if you've never had any experience with sports, you have all the skills necessary to lead this team. The way you handle the adversity is the way your family will ultimately handle it. Your attitude will spill over into theirs. Your determination is what will make things happen for your child, from your careful selection of their medical team, to being their voice and advocating for them. Sometimes that may mean trusting the doctor with a "third-string" reputation—he or she could be the superstar in your child's case!

After all, you are the only one who follows your child, day in and day out, through all matters, both medical and emotional, that relate to their condition. The doctors are there to direct you but ultimately, you are the final decision maker in your child's treatment. Sometimes you have to gather all the information and make the best possible decision based on your gut feeling. When dealing with JA you are often given choices in treatment, which can be very hard! Like a head coach, you must weigh those choices, consider the strengths and weaknesses of all the players, and make the *best* decisions for your child.

But, What About My Spouse?

Good question. If you are in a two-parent household, then of course both parents should be involved with all aspects of the child's treatment. However, there can only be one head coach. From the beginning, it's helpful if your family can approach the division of labor like a president and vice president. As much as you may try to share responsibilities, one parent always tends to be the primary caregiver. There should be one person in charge of organizing medical treatments, talking to doctors, dealing with insurance claims, etcetera, because it's so much more efficient and ensures nothing falls through the cracks.

This doesn't mean the other parent has a less important role. Both parents should attend doctor's appointments, whenever possible, and provide assistance in routine care for the child. The "other" parent should always be kept in the loop and included in all decision making;

however, having one parent be the point person will make everything run that much smoother.

Dividing up responsibilities becomes even more important when you have more than one child, as we do. When Grant required so much of my attention and had so many scheduled doctor appointments and therapies, my husband Fred could be available for Evan (who was undiagnosed and well at the time). Since I had been with Grant at all the appointments and I was also keeping the journal, it was easier for me to match the explanation of benefits (EOBs) from the insurance company with the bills from the hospital, and even catch errors. Also, since I was with Grant most of the time, if the doctor contacted us by phone or e-mail, I had a better feel for all the subtle changes and warning signs that he would show. I was the more efficient and accurate reporter of his true condition.

In the beginning, Fred did try to answer the calls from the doctor or insurance case manager, but found that many times his information was less complete than mine, because he wasn't there or didn't remember everything I had summarized (we tend to remember more when we actually do something than just hear about it). After a couple of omissions in communication, we decided it would be best to divide our duties a different way. It wasn't that I was more important than my husband—it was just that things really *did* work better with one head coach.

My husband is still involved in the improvements or digressions in Grant's case, but he doesn't have the pressure of knowing everything *all* of the time, or the need to regurgitate it on a moment's notice. He can focus his energies on other things and free me up in a different area (like managing school or sports). I also think the outside parties involved appreciate a streamlined communication process, which makes the whole situation easier to deal with.

Trusting Yourself

During one of Grant's inpatient admissions, we saw a new rheumatologist on rounds. Our "regular" rheumy (parental lingo for rheumatologist) was not at the hospital that day, and some things had happened overnight that left me with a million questions. As this new doctor patiently listened to my concerns, she answered what she could and then said "*You know, if you put 100 rheumatologists in the same room with the same kid, you would probably get 100 different treatment plans.*" That really hit home.

I had been a little down in the dumps about Grant's lack of progress and the fact that he had actually regressed some over the last few months. It seemed as though we no sooner got one problem under control than another related issue would pop up. When I was asking this rheumatologist so many questions, she kept referring back to his chart to see what his plan entailed. It confused me a little. Shouldn't she know what his plan was? Her response about the "100 different plans" explained why she kept referring back to his file—it was not only to review his case, but to review the unique treatment plan he was following. If he had been her patient, that plan could have been very different.

The Doctor Isn't Always Right

Although there are recognized protocols and typical plans of action, the way each rheumatologist can interpret each child's case and tweak that plan gives us an infinite number of possibilities—some very different and some only slightly so. It was an epiphany: I suddenly realized that if I was unhappy with the current plan, I had other options. I needed to talk to our regular doctor, tell her why I didn't think the plan was working, and see what else we could do. It seems pretty simple in retrospect, but at the time, I had no idea how much input we, as parents, could have on Grant's treatment plan and what an impact that could make.

The doctors had the medical training necessary to develop a course of action, something I could never do without them, but I had the most information about my child, how he reacted to medications, and how he responded to treatments. I knew my child best, and to get him the most beneficial care, I realized that day that the doctors needed me as much as I needed them.

This was a huge turning point for me as a parent. Looking back over Grant's entire case (from the age of two to the present time), I realized that the doctors aren't always right. They are human like the rest of us, with a very special area of expertise. They may be presented with an unfamiliar set of circumstances and be making educated guesses as well. I didn't have to go along with everything they said or told me to do— ultimately it was *our* call—a decision made together. Sometimes, I had to trust my gut and push to find answers for things that I knew just weren't right, despite reassurances that they were. Other times, I had to make a tough choice between drug options that were offered to my son, with side effects that I didn't want to face, or insist that we were seeing atypical side effects so his medications could be changed.

I learned to question their authority, but in a respectful way. I wished I had learned this lesson sooner! If I had trusted my instincts and refused his prescription of sulfa drugs (I was squeamish because I have a severe sulfa allergy and Grant had never taken them), he never would have been hospitalized with DRESS syndrome. Don't get me wrong, in that case the prescribing doctor did not do anything wrong, and we don't blame her. All her logic in prescribing the drug was solid, according to proven medical protocols. A parent's allergy doesn't guarantee the child's. It was the most effective drug with the least side effects, and she started slowly, to check for a reaction. Grant reacted atypically, and very late, so there was no way to know ... but I *should* have trusted my mommy gut!

Sometimes, the doctor's hands are tied, based on the particular hospital protocols. The first time Grant had inter-articular joint injections, it was with a drug that is known to have a fairly short period of relief. That was the only drug available for this purpose at that particular hospital. The following year, the same hospital approved the use of a different drug by request that lasted three times longer! When I asked around, I discovered that some other children's hospitals were using the longer-acting drug on a regular basis, several years prior to our hospital's use. When I realized that the drugs my child could have access to might depend on the system to which the doctor belonged, we sought out a second opinion from another clinic with a completely different set of protocols. I didn't "ditch" Grant's primary team, but a fresh set of eyes, with a different opinion and an alternate set of choices, appealed to us. We wanted to have all options available to him and follow whatever plan would work the best in his unique case.

About a year after my epiphany, I was questioning the doctors more. I had a few areas of concern that didn't seem to worry the doctors much. Since Grant had been given large amounts of corticosteroids and taken almost a year to wean off of them, he had gained an excessive amount of weight, which is fairly typical. He had also grown very little, if at all over the same time period. Limited growth can also be a side effect of steroids and the high levels of inflammation he had been experiencing. As a middle school student, the lack of growth and excess weight were very problematic for Grant. He looked so different that, one day while I was in the pick-up line at the school reading a book, he actually startled me when he got in the car. For a minute, it didn't register that he was my kid! He would tell me often that when he looked in the mirror, he didn't even see himself anymore. The changes were that drastic.

Around that time, I began to research steroids a little more and talk with other parents. I had a sinking feeling that more was going on than just the aftereffects of steroids. It was taking too long. His diet was great, he was exercising, and his flares were getting further apart, so why weren't we seeing positive changes in his weight or growth? Even after approaching a few of his specialists several times, I was assured that it was nothing to worry about, but I was still worried. My gut told me differently, and I continued to question them (I had learned my lesson). When his pediatrician recognized how much it was affecting Grant emotionally and knowing how long I had been concerned, he agreed to help us rule out some other possibilities.

With autoimmune diseases, so many systems can be affected that it could be plausible to see almost every specialist in the book. Part of caring for your child is finding balance. Early on, I think we didn't start seeing an endocrinologist because we couldn't be sure that Grant had a problem in that area, and we didn't want to overwhelm him with more doctors or spend *all* of his time in a clinic. His pediatrician knew the first few things that an endocrinologist would need to determine if there was a growth disorder. He ordered two bone age tests, six months apart, and when they came back with little change, he helped us get in to see an endocrinologist right away.

The endocrinologist confirmed my suspicions. Grant had a significant growth hormone deficiency that was causing the lack of growth and could be partially responsible for the excess weight. The lack of growth hormone could also affect his ability to heal—not a great scenario for someone whose body was attacking itself! Since Grant was already 12 and had limited years to grow, time was of the essence. His endocrinologist was instrumental in getting the medications he needed approved through our insurance, and we had high hopes that we would see positive changes soon.

Six months later, his growth looked great, but the weight issue hadn't changed. Using my trusty journal, I explained to the endocrinologist what types of food he was eating and how much. I had also kept track of his exercise and sleep. Everything should have pointed to improved weight loss. She listened and then ordered a simple test that revealed that Grant had insulin resistance, a possible precursor to autoimmune diabetes. Without help in this area, he wasn't going to lose any more weight, period. She tweaked his medications, added another, and within just a few weeks, my son was back to his old self. He was sleeping better, had more energy, and, best of all, was happy again. If I had just accepted what I was told in the beginning, we would have lost valuable time, or even developed another issue. Eventually, I believe the other doctors would have realized something else was wrong, but I am grateful that I stood my ground, kept pushing, and had an amazing pediatrician to back me up and take my concerns seriously.

GRASPING AT STRAWS (EMI'S STORY) by AMBER

When the Red Cross message came through, one line stood out from the rest: "possible loss of life." As I read in disbelief, I thought "*What if I never get to see my baby again?*" I had been on a deployment in the Middle East, and although I knew my five-year-old daughter, Emi, was ill, I had no idea how severe her condition was until that moment. At that point, my only mission was to get home.

While I was traveling halfway around the world, Emi was lying in the hospital. My husband and I talked twice a day, usually during the doctor's rounds, so he could answer my growing list of questions. Google was my lifeline. Before we received a definitive diagnosis, the doctor mentioned Still's disease, which I immediately began to research. As I read the description, I remember thinking it sounded very serious and hoping the doctor was wrong. As it turns out, Still's disease is another name for systemic onset juvenile idiopathic arthritis (SOJIA). In my opinion, the term Still's disease does a better job of describing this condition, because "arthritis" downplays the severity.

When I walked into Emi's hospital room on that first night after arriving home, I was shocked. She was pale and lethargic, sleeping most of the day and night, and was too tired to even whine or complain. Her fever was troubling. The next day, Emi was started on a nonsteroid anti-inflammatory (NSAID), which finally brought the fever down. After 24 hours without a fever, she was released from the hospital. Though still ill, it had been determined that it was "just arthritis," and we were referred to a rheumatologist.

Since it was close to Easter and I was only supposed to be home for two weeks, we decided to decorate eggs and have a little fun. But our little celebration didn't last long. Emi's fever returned that night and this time it reached a high of 104.6. The fever became episodic: She would spike a fever twice a day for two to four hours and become completely lethargic, and then it would subside. During one of these episodes, as I lay in bed next to her, Emi rolled over and vomited before returning to sleep. Normally she hates being wet and dirty, but she didn't even seem to notice. That's when I knew something was terribly wrong.

We returned to the doctor's office the next day and conveyed our concerns about the first rheumatology appointment still being two days away. More blood work was ordered, which revealed that Emi was suddenly anemic. This news pushed up our appointment with the rheumatologist, so we hurried off to another hospital.

Because Emi's symptoms were "atypical" (i.e., there was no joint involvement) the rheumatologist would not begin treatment until she ran a new battery of tests, including a bone marrow biopsy and spinal tap—everything else had to be ruled out. Meanwhile, in less than 24 hours, Emi had become so anemic that she required a blood transfusion. Once the test results came back, we were sent by ambulance to the children's hospital. They had confirmed that she had SOJIA, and it was getting bad, fast.

On that first night in the children's hospital, the attending pediatrician told me she would be right outside our room all night and to let her know immediately if Emi's condition seemed to get worse. In my mind, I decided I was the first responder here. If Emi's heart stopped and the doctors didn't get in her room fast enough, I would begin CPR. Never in a million years did I think I would make a parenting decision of that magnitude, and yet here I was.

The next day we were transferred to the ICU. The SOJIA was causing inflammation around her heart and lungs, and possibly her brain. The doctors began giving Emi pulse steroids, interleukin-1 inhibitor injections, acid reducers, more NSAIDs and taking daily blood work. Eventually, the fever resolved and her heart and lungs began to clear up.

This is when we were introduced to "roid rage" in a five-year-old. Emi hadn't had a tantrum since she turned four, but after two days on steroids, she launched herself into a four-hour fit of kicking and screaming. We were told that only time would resolve these super tantrums.

Despite this reaction to the steroids, we were feeling hopeful and expected to be discharged by the end of the week. After all, we had a diagnosis, she was on the proper medicine, and should be getting better, right? But Emi's fever returned. It crept back slowly and it was me who noticed the rise in temperature just by holding her. Another day of pulse steroids was ordered, and that's when the rash appeared. What started off as a scattering of tiny red bumps turned into an angry raised mass that spread across her torso. The rash would come and go along with the fever, leaving her exhausted but unable to sleep. This was something new. Emi had macrophage activation syndrome (MAS), a life-threatening complication of rheumatic disease.

Even after reading as much as I could about MAS, I still had no idea what it was. I did, however, understand one thing—it had a 20 percent mortality rate! Once it was diagnosed, Emi was given cyclosporine, which caused vomiting. She couldn't eat, drink or hold down any of her medicine, so everything went through her IV. To make matters worse, her inflammation numbers kept climbing, which mystified the rheumatologist.

After a week on IV cyclosporine and pulse steroids the numbers marking inflammation in her blood finally began to drop and the fever went away. The rash has always mocked us though. It comes and goes, usually only lasting 30 minutes to an hour, and sometimes we only notice because suddenly Emi is very itchy. It's something we've learned to live with—a reminder that there is no cure for this disease, only control.

Once her numbers were looking good, about three weeks after being admitted to the children's hospital and five weeks into her total hospital stay, the doctor suggested oral steroids. I had a horrible feeling about this course of treatment for several reasons. But we seemed to have no other options. Emi needed to get home and to do that we had to be completely off IV medication.

The doctor thought the steroids would be absorbed better if we doubled the oral dose, so Emi began taking a dose of steroids usually prescribed for someone four times her weight. Twenty four hours and two doses into this treatment her stomach suddenly swelled up, becoming huge and taut. Within the next fifteen minutes, she was screaming in pain. You know things are bad when five doctors suddenly appear in the room and a surgery consult is requested. I learned it was possible for her intestines to rip, which allows feces to leak into the body—a serious problem when your immune system is suppressed.

Thankfully, it was only an ileus—her bowels had temporarily shut down from all the stress and possibly the medication. Emi received a gastrointestinal (GI) tube and was fed a liquid diet for the next two days. During this time, three different rheumatologists examined Emi and all of them had their own take on her treatment. One doctor mentioned to me that she would have *never* allowed Emi to take such high dosages of oral steroids. It was this comment that made me realize that these doctors, while trained, were grasping at treatment straws. They were making educated guesses about Emi's treatment, and in some cases, they were wrong. SOJIA is not the same for every child, and it's extremely rare for this condition to make a child as sick as Emi.

In total, Emi spent 57 days in the hospital, including two weeks in the ICU. When she was discharged, she was so weak that she couldn't even stand up without help. She was also terribly sad. In addition to her weekly visit to rheumatology, we took her to physical therapy, occupational therapy, and a psychologist. She is now on bi-weekly infusions, a small dose of oral steroids, cyclosporine and an acid reducer, and is doing much better, although she has more joint problems now. To be honest, it still feels like a guessing game.

Still, we are grateful because Emi is home with us and happy again. Throughout this experience, we've learned a great deal. We've learned to parent all over again because parenting a chronically ill child has its own challenges. We've learned to focus on teaching her to live with this disease, so Emi is learning to swim, which helps her stay in shape and is easy on the joints. Though she may be in pain, we stress the importance of not using her condition as a reason not to do things. We've learned that doctors are not always right, and that sometimes you have to trust your gut instinct. Most of all, we've learned to be thankful for every good day.

Consider ALL Your Sources

The truth is, it's impossible for any doctor to provide all the answers. This disease is very complex, different for every child, and varied in every situation. The doctors are good at what they do, but they can only do so much. Sometimes you have to fill in the blanks from other sources.

The first time Grant was hospitalized, it took him a very long time to bounce back. He was exhausted and weak, and he spent much of his time at the clinic and the hospital as an outpatient for tests and labs. When his lab work started coming back with better results, his rheumatologist encouraged us to get him back into school full time as soon as possible. Since keeping mobile is a big part of controlling the negative effects of JA, her advice seemed reasonable, but Grant told me he just wasn't ready.

About a week into trying to survive a normal day at school, Grant's principal gave me a call. His teachers agreed—Grant was not ready to come back into a full-time school environment. He was falling down frequently and having a difficult time concentrating. His medications still made him feel ill, and despite efforts on everyone's part, he wasn't getting very much out of his classes. It was obvious that he was stoically enduring high levels of pain, and sitting for such long periods of time didn't help matters. He frequently broke out in several different types of rashes and even had episodes with fever. He was fatigued to the point of complete exhaustion, and if he did stay at school all day, he could barely stay awake long enough to eat his dinner at home. It was too much. Grant knew it, and the school confirmed it. Once again, I was veering away from the doctor's advice, but she didn't get to see the whole picture.

I knew it was important to have Grant return to his normal life as soon as possible; he needed that normalcy not only to get well, but also to feel well. The concerns and advice the rheumatologist gave were valid, but Grant just wasn't ready for what his labs indicated he should be. His teachers knew him very well. After all, they spent almost eight hours a day with him, five days a week! They knew his personality, what he was capable of, and when he was trying to just get by. During the school year (before he was so seriously ill), they spent more waking hours with him than I did.

His teachers told me we needed a new plan. They didn't offer any advice about his medical situation, but their input regarding his daily life was invaluable. Under their recommendations, we modified Grant's work to the bare minimums. He kept the same scope and learned the same material as his peers, but his assignment load was reduced. He stopped going to regular classes and was assigned a homebound instructor who worked with him 1–3 hours a day, depending on how well he was feeling. The administration worked hard to allow him to come in for lunch, social events, and enrichment classes as he started feeling better, so he wouldn't be so disconnected from his peers.

By the end of the year, he had worked up to half days and was thriving. His stress levels were down, he was getting better, and he felt better, not overdone. His teachers knew just how hard to push to keep him honest and "normal" without making the situation worse. We were very lucky to have such a great team of educators and, without following *their* plan, I have no doubt that Grant's recovery would have taken much longer. As the head coach, I took my quarterback's read—the guy in the trenches (his teacher) over my offensive coordinator (the guy up in the booth, his doctor)—on this particular play. Those can be tough calls, but as long as you are making them with your head, armed with information from your *entire* team and not just based on emotion, chances are it will be the right call.

CHAPTER SIX

Controlling JA and Handling Flares

Juvenile arthritis has no cure. When my son was first diagnosed, I found that fact difficult to accept. In these days of medical miracles, it seemed unbelievable to me that so much is still unknown about this condition. Knowing that a cure was not yet in sight, our focus quickly turned to *how can we control this disease?* Current treatment plans center on reducing inflammation, relieving pain, preventing damage, and maximizing the child's ability to live a "normal" life. By working with your child's doctors and support staff, as well as other key players such as counselors, therapists, and educators, you will develop the best course of action for your child.

Medication

Central to any treatment plan for JA are the medications used to control the disease. In order to determine which medications are most effective, the doctor may require laboratory tests to identify the specific type of JA from which your child is suffering. Common tests include:

Anti-cyclic citrullinated peptide (anti-CCP) antibodies are used to help predict the possibility of undifferentiated arthritis developing into rheumatoid arthritis.

Rheumatoid factor (RF) measures the presence of an autoantibody, although rare in JA. (An autoantibody is a type of protein manufactured by the immune system that is directed against one or more of the body's own proteins.)

Antinuclear antibody (ANA) measures the presence of an autoantibody against the cells' nuclei, which can help narrow diagnosis and alert the doctor to an increased risk for eye disease.

Erythrocyte sedimentation rate (ESR) is the rate at which red blood cells drop to the bottom of the test tube, which can help indicate whether inflammation is present.

C-reactive protein (CRP) measures the presence of an acute-phase protein produced in the liver. When levels of CRP rise in the blood, it is often an indicator of increased inflammation. Although its purpose is similar to the ESR test, it is a different way to measure inflammation.

X-rays, MRIs, and additional laboratory tests may be used to rule out or confirm other underlying issues or to provide a baseline for future reference.

Once the doctor has a better feel for the type of JA with which you are dealing, the medications that may be prescribed usually fall into one of four categories:

Nonsteroidal anti-inflammatory drugs (NSAIDs) Often the first type of medication used, NSAIDs help reduce inflammation and pain. Many NSAIDs are available over the counter (OTC), but some subclasses, including COX-2 inhibitors, are available only by prescription. Keep in mind, just because a drug is available without a prescription does not mean it won't cause side effects or interact adversely with other medications. It's very important to keep your child's doctor informed of *any* OTC medications that are being used and to watch for potential side effects. In addition, long-term use of any drug requires monitoring by a medical professional. Some children respond better to one NSAID over another, so careful observation of your child can help his/her doctor find the "right" fit.

Disease-modifying antirheumatic drugs (DMARDs) If NSAIDs are not sufficient, DMARDs will often be prescribed. This type of drug slows the progression of the disease, but can take weeks or months to be fully effective. Although there are several types of DMARDs, the most common type prescribed to children with JA is methotrexate, which can be administered via pill or injection. **Corticosteroids** Usually used in severe cases or during a flare, corticosteroids such as prednisone are used to reduce inflammation quickly. Administration can be done orally or intravenously. Steroids offer considerable benefits, but also come with many undesirable side effects, such as significant weight gain, "moon" face, weakened bones, and stunted growth. In some cases, steroids can mean the difference between life and death. For this reason, it's critical to follow doctor's orders in their administration, although many parents are hesitant to use them due to the side effects. Since it can be dangerous to stop steroids suddenly, it's just as important to follow your doctor's directions in tapering off these medications as it is to begin their administration. If few joints are affected and there is no systemic necessity for their use, steroids may also be injected directly into an affected joint (inter-articular joint injections) to provide relief without systemic side effects. **Biologic agents** are one of the newest classes of treatments, also known as biologic response modifiers. Some biologics are tumor necrosis factor (TNF) inhibitors. TNF is a naturally occurring protein that causes inflammation. Other biologics work slightly differently, blocking inflammatory T-cells, or interleukin-1, another distinct inflammatory protein.

TIPS FOR "SHOT NIGHT"

Administering shots at home is a big deal. No kid likes receiving them and no parent enjoys giving them! Add the fear of doing it wrong into the mix and shot night can turn into stress night. Here are a few of the tricks we've learned along the way to make shot night a little less stressful.

1. Get the training. Whether it's from the drug company nurse who is sent to your home to train you, or the nurse in your child's doctor's office, take advantage of the training and information they can provide. Even if *you* are a nurse, it's different with your own child (or at least that's what my nurse friends tell me!), and there may be specific information about the drug or delivery system that could help make your administration run smoother.

2. Make sure the vial is at room or body temperature. Many of the injectable drugs for JA must be stored in the refrigerator, but cold medication can make the injection more painful. Be sure to check with the doctor or pharmacist first, but most medications can be taken out of the fridge 30–45 minutes in advance and warmed by holding it in your hand a few minutes before injecting. The closer the liquid is to body temperature, the less painful it seems to be. Some moms swear by the "bra method" warming the vial between their skin and bra until it no longer feels cold. This ensures that you don't leave the vial out too long, and still allows you to move about doing other chores, but we have had equal success leaving the medication out on the counter, setting a timer and warming it slightly in our hands prior to injection.

3. Prep the area properly. Prior to administering the shot, it's important to sterilize the area. Alcohol wipes are normally the preferred method, but they can sting. Make sure to allow a few extra seconds for the alcohol to evaporate and dry *before* the injection; or ask the doctor if an alternative method (like washing with surgical soap) could be considered. In our case, we found the soap and water method to be more comfortable, and the liquid surgical soap is readily available as an over-the-counter purchase through our local pharmacy. A quick swipe with a saturated sterile cotton ball followed by a swipe with a damp cotton ball to rinse is the method we prefer.

4. Know and prepare your child. Prepping him or her mentally for the shot is different for every child. Some kids need advance notice, or like to be included in the decisions, such as choosing the injection site or which day of the week will be "the" night. Others would prefer not to anticipate the shot and get it over with as quickly as possible. Reducing your child's stress prior to the injection will help to increase their comfort levels.

5. Utilize pain management techniques. Depending on the medication, some injections are very painful, while others are only mildly uncomfortable. In either case, there are several steps that can be taken to reduce discomfort. Buzzy (www.buzzy4shots.com) is a product system designed by a doctor that has been clinically proven to reduce pain for injections, intravenous placement, and blood draws. We have had quite a bit of success with this product, but some of its effects can be replicated using a combination of ice for several minutes on the injection site, along with a handheld massager to numb the area and confuse the nerves.

6. Provide distraction. Watching something funny or engaging on television can help divert the focus, while decreasing stress and the sensation of pain. One strange but effective tip (for older children) we picked up from a hematology/oncology nurse was to pop a very sour hard candy in Grant's mouth, right at the time of injection. The brain focuses so much on the "sour" sensation that the needle prick becomes secondary.

7. Provide positive reinforcement. When things go well, don't forget to brag on your child, letting him or her know how proud you are. Some parents provide a reward system, such as a star on the calendar or a small treat, while others offer only verbal praise. Again, use whatever system works for your family, but don't forget to recognize your child for good compliance and bravery.

Physical, Occupational, and Alternative Therapies

In addition to drug therapies, your child may be prescribed a course of physical and/or occupational therapy. Physical therapy (PT) can help maintain or increase range of motion in affected joints. The physical therapist or rehabilitation specialist can also help design an exercise program that is appropriate for your child's age and level of disease involvement. Regular exercise is a very important component of the treatment plan. It will help decrease pain and stiffness, while preserving mobility and muscle tone—and it's not just a series of boring exercises anymore! Pediatric physical therapists have many tricks up their sleeves to make sessions fun and more play-like. Alternate forms of physical therapy, including water/aquatic therapy and hippotherapy (done on horseback), can provide a change of routine that children may enjoy and are often covered by insurance as well.

When JA gets in the way of normal daily functions, occupational therapy (OT) may be indicated. OT can help your child by making adjustments to his/her home and school environment, as well as teaching the child to make modifications so he or she can participate in more activities. Many times, occupational therapy also trains parents and children in the use of adaptive equipment that will help them obtain their goals.

Another component of your child's treatment plan might include complementary and alternative therapies. Many of these treatments, including chiropractic care, acupuncture, massage, diet and nutritional supplements, are gaining approval in the mainstream medical community and may help alleviate some symptoms. In fact, several insurance carriers are beginning to cover these therapies, especially if a practitioner who meets their defined criteria administers them. However, **before undertaking any complementary or alternative medication or therapy it's critical that the medical team is onboard with the proposed treatment.** If your child's doctor doesn't feel it will do any harm or interact negatively with the current course of treatment, then it's safe to proceed. Even over-the-counter vitamins or certain foods can cause issues with some medications, so it's important to make your medical team aware of *everything* that is included in your child's treatment plan. In the long run, this will also help the medical team determine what works and what doesn't work in your child's individual case. Even if your doctor is not opposed to a particular alternative treatment, they may prefer to introduce it at another time, so they can adequately evaluate a different part of the plan. For instance, if you change your child's diet *and* alter medication at the same time, it's difficult to determine which change, or if either, was helpful.

When progress is slow, it's tempting to take matters into your own hands, but it's not the best idea for your child. You may be the head coach, but you can't play the game alone! Always communicate with your child's doctor and make changes (if any) based on your mutual decisions.

Don't Forget Routine Care

Now that your child may be seeing a long list of specialists and therapists due to JA, it's easy to put routine care on the back burner. After all, who wants to see another doctor? Still, keeping in touch with your pediatrician to make sure all the normal well-child care stays up to date is important. Likewise, be sure to schedule regular appointments with your child's dentist. In addition to routine care, the dentist can also watch for progression of JA in the jaw or inadequate oral hygiene due to joint pain in the hands. If your child previously suffered from another chronic condition (such as allergies or asthma), make sure the course of treatment for the other condition is being followed and complements the plan for JA. Allowing any of these other ailments to "slide" could make things much more complicated in the long run.

Consider Counseling

We've talked quite a bit about preserving the physical functioning of your child through various medications and therapies, but that is only part of the picture. Mental health plays a large role in your child's quality of life, and counseling may be necessary in order to help your child cope with all the changes and challenges of JA. Accepting the diagnosis, dealing with depression, and developing coping mechanisms are important elements of your child's treatment.

Sometimes working with a professional is more effective than hearing it from mom or dad, and there is no shame in seeing a mental health professional. Seeking help is not a weakness, and if there is a "good fit" with a counselor, then you may find your child actually enjoying the sessions. In some cases, having yet another doctor appointment may be just too much. When my son was experiencing medical burnout, the counseling sessions were the first thing he was ready to cut out. He didn't feel he needed them, and they took time away from his friends and down time (which was already scarce). However, I still felt he needed to be able to talk out his problems with a trained professional outside the family. We compromised on his school social worker, who could be accessed during school hours, and who agreed to alert us if he needed to seek more extensive help. Regardless, it is always good to have an objective opinion on your child's mental health during these extraordinarily difficult times. (For more on finding support for your child, see chapter 11.)

Specialists, medications, therapies, counseling … I know it seems overwhelming! At some point, however, you will have it all figured out (I promise it happens!). Those are great times, but they typically don't last forever. Eventually, everything will get turned upside down all over again—that's when you find yourself dealing with a flare.

Handling Flares

Just when you think you have things under control (as much as can be expected anyway) your child may experience a flare. Basically a *flare* is any increase in symptoms beyond your child's normal baseline. Flares can be very disruptive, painful, and even frightening. They can rob your child (and you) of regular rest and make normal activities almost impossible. But they might not. Sometimes a flare comes on hard and fast, leaving you no time to prepare; other times there are warning signs that a flare is eminent, allowing you to treat it quickly and reduce the severity. It all depends on your child and the circumstances.

Exactly one year after Grant's first hospitalization, he had a very serious flare that landed him in the hospital again. His fever spiked to well over 104 degrees and was accompanied by a rash, excruciating pain, and hot swollen joints. One of his arms swelled to nearly twice its normal size! It was a scary time, as nothing we did at home was alleviating his symptoms.

At the opposite end of the spectrum, there have been instances, often on the heels of a cold or virus, when we have observed warning signs, such as an increase in Grant's episcleritis (irritation and inflammation of the thin layer of tissue covering the white part of the eye) and a slight change in joint comfort. Knowing that a flare may be coming allowed us to consult with the doctor, tweak his medications, and avert a full episode. However, most times his flares have been somewhere in the middle, ranging from a few days to a few weeks of increased symptoms. Each time, the doctors have helped us change the game plan to get his symptoms back under control.

Our Bag of Tricks

When dealing with a flare, the first thing we always worry about is getting a handle on Grant's discomfort. In addition to working with the doctors to adjust his medications and attack the root of the problem, there are other things that can be done to alleviate the symptoms. If the flare is severe enough, the answer may be hospitalization. If it's serious, but doesn't require a hospital visit, life usually comes to a halt while we focus on everything we can to make things bearable for him. Sleep and rest become priorities, and all schedules are thrown out the window.

Sometimes the side effects from the medications can be as bad as the flare itself, trading one set of issues (pain, fever, swelling) for another (nausea, headaches, fatigue). In our family, we pull out the special bag of tricks, just for this occasion—all doctor approved, of course! Warm baths, cool compresses, alternating heat with cold on swollen joints, and dimly lit rooms may help. Some find that aromatherapy can be helpful as well, with lavender or another soothing scent added to the room or bath.

For a moderate flare, we may do all of those things as well as add some distraction. Laughter can be the best medicine. Did you know that at UCLA, the Pediatric Pain Program and the Jonsson Comprehensive Cancer Center did a joint research project to prove that laughter can reduce pain and increase healing in sick children? Now known as "Rx Laughter," results from the study indicated that children exposed to humor experienced less anxiety and pain when dealing with painful medical procedures. Adults reported sleeping better and having less pain as well. College students that were studied showed fewer respiratory infections among those who laughed more often—and laughter is *not* counter-indicated with any drug! I used to say that if standing on my head and singing "Yankee Doodle Dandy" would work to reduce Grant's pain, I would do it. Now there is solid evidence that it just might help after all! If nothing else, laughter breaks the monotony of staying home sick and improves mental and emotional health.

Although your child may not be up for any strenuous activity or able to focus in school, a favorite movie or television show can take their mind off things just enough to alleviate some symptoms and fight the boredom of staying home a few days. We also use these periods to catch up on one-on-one time, play a board game, or just talk. This is also one of the few times that I ease up on video game restrictions. If the flare is bad enough, and it helps distract him, then some rules are tabled until later.

This doesn't mean I allow a "free ride" with every flare. Some flares have been mild enough that Grant could push himself through the academic periods at school and come home to rest during the "special" or non-academic periods. During a mild flare, being at school with a purpose and visiting with his friends not only kept him feeling "normal" and up-to-date with schoolwork, but also provided a productive distraction from milder pain. Knowing what type of flare you are dealing with and knowing what your child needs without pushing too hard or allowing too much latitude is the name of the game. In time, you will become a pro at figuring out what works and when.

PREPARING FOR A FLARE

Flares can be unpredictable—coming on at anytime, anywhere. However, by planning ahead, you can be prepared to handle the situation.

1. At home, make sure you have all your supplies handy. In our house, no one drinks the last ginger ale! If anyone has significant nausea, I know there is at least *one* ginger ale and some fresh saltines to tide us over until a store run can be made. Also, never let your prescriptions run down too low, because during a flare your doctor may have you temporarily increase the dosage or change the mix of medications. If your child is hurting and in need, the last thing you want to do is run around obtaining things that could already be helping them feel better.

2. Have a meeting with your child's teacher and the school nurse to discuss what a flare could look like in your child. Have a plan in place that will allow the school nurse to administer medication or allow your child to rest in her office if necessary, as well as guidelines for missing school and making up work.

3. Even if your child has been doing well, be ready for the worst, especially when traveling. Before leaving on a trip, let your doctors know so they may be more available via email or phone for questions that may arise when you're unable to be seen. Find out which nearby hospitals would best suit your child's needs, should an inpatient admission become necessary. Always travel with your prescriptions, and call the pharmacy in advance if a refill will be needed outside your home territory, as some drugs need a longer lead time for ordering. Check with your insurance to see what process you need to follow in order to have medical services covered outside your home area. Finally, even though it's extra "stuff" to pack, don't forget all the comfort items your child uses during a flare, including heating pads, gel ice packs, handheld massagers, etc.

CHAPTER SEVEN

Pain Management

It was 3:47 a.m. I remember because the clock was flashing and I was coming out of a deep sleep, still groggy and trying to get my bearings. Grant's hand was on my shoulder, gently shaking me awake as he leaned over and supported himself on my bed.

"Mom?" he murmured in the dark.

The last few days had been really hard on all of us. Grant's pain levels had been so high that no one was getting any real sleep, emotions were raw, and we were starting to feel more than a little desperate. Nothing seemed to be working to alleviate his discomfort, and it was wearing on all of us. On that particular night, I couldn't believe I had scored such a long stretch of sleep, until he spoke again, his words hitting me like a punch to the gut: "I tried to wait as long as I could to get you," he whispered, so as not to wake his dad. "I haven't gone to sleep yet—it hurts *so* bad." It took me a moment to process the information: *It was almost 4 a.m. and he hadn't slept yet?*

"I'm so sorry, Mom," he continued. "I know you need your rest, so I waited as long as I could, but I just can't do it anymore. I need your help. Is there **anything** you can do to make it **any** better? I could barely walk in here to get you on my own …"

It was all I could do to fight back the tears. It just wasn't fair. Grant was barely 11 years old and too young to be dealing with such horrible chronic pain; yet he was worried about *me*. I told him to lie down in my spot, while I prepared a warm bath in our whirlpool tub and headed downstairs to the kitchen to get him a little snack. Since it was already early morning, his pain medications from the night before had worn off. Even though the meds didn't seem to be doing much for him, I knew that letting them lapse would make it that much harder to get on top of the pain again. I never thought I would sleep that long.

As I padded downstairs (silently cursing myself for not setting an alarm and feeling guilty that he had been going through this alone all night), I tried to think what would make a good snack—one that wouldn't interfere with his bath, but would put enough in his stomach so the meds I was about to give him wouldn't make him sick. My brain was already going 100 miles per hour. I settled on half a piece of toast, with a little cream cheese, and a juice glass filled with sparkling water. I also pulled a cold pack out of the freezer.

I made my way upstairs, still clumsy from not enough sleep, and struggling to carry everything up without spilling. A big part of me hoped I had prepared this snack for nothing; that I would find him fast asleep in my place, getting a little relief—an escape through slumber. I would gladly take the remainder of the night banished to the couch, tossing the toast, and wasting the water in the tub, but I knew I wouldn't be that lucky.

As I came down the hall, I could hear my son whimpering softly and groaning when the next wave of pain hit him. Though I was expecting it, my heart sank anyway. This was my stoic child—the one who never cried when he got a shot, not even as a toddler, the one who other parents would marvel at being the "toughest" kid on the football team. If he was moaning now, it *had* to be bad. And since I hadn't even entered the room yet, I knew his sounds of distress were not just for attention.

Grant was wide awake, just as I knew he would be. His back and ankles were so hot, it felt like he was running a fever, but just on those spots. He reached for the cold pack as soon as I got close. "I'll do this now," he said. "Because it works even though I hate it."

I finished filling the tub, dimmed the lights, and perched the plate with his snack and pills on the side of the tub so he could take his meds as soon as possible—call it "bathtub multitasking" if you will. When I called him in, Grant asked me if I could help him into the tub, and if he could wear his shorts in the water, so I could just stay with him. Normally, it's nice to feel needed, but under these circumstances, it was the worst feeling ever.

Feeling Helpless

Over the next few years, I had that emotion a lot. Words cannot begin to describe the helplessness I have felt when my child is experiencing excruciating pain and there is absolutely nothing to be done. Being a parent of children with JIA is difficult, but for me, dealing with their pain is definitely the hardest component.

When Grant was so ill that we didn't know what the future held for him, I felt as though I was moving around in a fog—a dreamlike state where none of it seemed real. We kept going through the motions, but we were shell-shocked and numb. Lucky for us, that time passed fairly quickly, although many other families are not so fortunate and have a different experience. Those periods were difficult in their own way, but we had so many things to process and so much to do that we didn't have much time to sit and worry, or feel sorry for ourselves. The pain issue is completely different. When your child is hurting and there is nothing you can do except to observe the suffering, it's like time stands still. For a parent, that is pure torture.

When most people hear about arthritis, they think of aches and pains. It can be that, but it can also be far more serious. Grant's pain was so relentless that he didn't sleep through the night uninterrupted for more than a year. Severe discomfort would wake him from a sound slumber. Though he took some medications for pain and others to assist him with sleep, it still wasn't enough for him to lead a "normal" life. Sometimes he couldn't even make it out of bed or to the restroom without help. At its most intense, the pain would cause his legs to buckle underneath him and he would nearly pass out. Extreme or prolonged pain can, at times, be too much for the body to handle. When this occurs, the pain is often "referred" to other areas of the body where nothing is wrong. In addition to this type of referred pain, Grant would sometimes experience nausea, headaches, and all-over achiness. It kept him from being able to focus in school, participate in activities with his friends, or be an average kid. It made me feel helpless.

More than Physical

Although it's a very intense experience wondering if your child may live or die, it's equally traumatic to hear your preteen say he is no longer sure he *wants* to live, because he just can't take hurting so much anymore. I remember that time like it was yesterday. Grant was 12 years old and doing time as an inpatient again. We were watching TV, feeling a little bored, when he turned to me and said matter-of-factly, "It would be okay if I pass away the next time things get really bad ... not that I want to kill myself or anything, but because at least then I'll be in heaven and it won't hurt anymore. It would be okay, Mom. It's not like I'll ever have my real life back anyway."

His words took my breath away. I wanted more than anything to remove this burden from him. I would have gladly taken it in his place. It's a hard thing for a parent to know that your child may feel this way, not due to teenage angst or suicidal thoughts, but because they are just so worn out from pain they can never escape.

Although the damage that can occur with JIA is a major concern to parents, the issue that haunts many of us is the pain. No parent wants to see their child hurting, especially on a daily basis. Chronic pain is very draining emotionally and physically on the entire family. Even siblings are not untouched by the suffering. In the early days, I had to insist that my boys *not* share a room as they had their entire lives, because I found Grant was disrupting Evan's sleep. Although he was only in the fourth grade, if Evan was awakened by Grant's restlessness, he would often stay up with him for a good portion of the night, making sure he was okay, or getting him a hot or cold pack without my knowledge. He wanted to make it better, too, and felt the same helplessness we all experienced.

The pain from JA can range from a nagging irritation to a completely debilitating condition that brings daily life to an abrupt halt. It can change from one to the other at the drop of a dime, so even if the pain is minor, it's like an elephant in the room. Everyone knows it's there, and we all hold our breath in the hopes it won't stampede and make everything much worse.

In order to effectively deal with your child's pain, it's important to understand it. Pain can be physical, psychological, or both. Regardless of the type, the pain is real, and even though it may feel hopeless, there *are* things you can do.

Getting Help

Pain may be an issue that children with JA are faced with frequently, but it should *not* be something they "just live with." Pain is a sign of something: It's the body's way of alerting you that all is not right. If pain levels change dramatically, it's important to find out why and what may have altered to cause the difference.

The First Line of Defense—Your Pediatrician

At the risk of sounding like a broken record, I will say it again: Contact your pediatrician first. Let him/her know what is going on and ask for their input. Pediatricians can examine the whole child, without the prejudice of a specialty, and help point you in the right direction. By now, you will probably have developed a pretty good relationship with your pediatrician, and he or she will also have a feel for your child's mental state to help determine if that's a contributing factor.

After Grant had been diagnosed for some time and Evan was new in his diagnosis, Evan started complaining of severe heel pain. It was getting bad enough that any more than two or three blocks of walking caused him to wince in pain and limp. I had checked his shoes; they were high quality and still fitting properly, and he had no injuries of which to speak.

Since Grant had arthritis in *his* subtalar joints (where the heel meets the ankle) and it was serious enough to warrant inter-articular steroid injections, you can imagine what conclusion I was jumping to! After all, Evan already had a JIA diagnosis, even though we had only seen involvement in his elbows and fingers to date. My first thought was that his disease was progressing and affecting more joints, and if I had taken him straight to the rheumatologist, given his history, that may have been the consensus. Rather than self-diagnose or utilize the rheumatologist just yet, I e-mailed our pediatrician.

We had noticed the pain for about a week and it was getting worse. I knew how fast these things can get away from you, so I was relieved he was willing to see us on short notice (it's wonderful to have such a great, caring doctor). After the exam, a good talk, and a few heel squeezes, he was open to the thought that Evan's pain could be JA, but had a suspicion it might be Sever's disease instead. Although that sounds scary, it's actually a fairly common issue during periods of high growth, where the joint can't quite keep up with the rapid changes and becomes inflamed. Often, with rest, anti-inflammatory medication, and the use of heel cups in the shoes, the condition will go away in just a few weeks. Since the pain was bearable, we tried that approach before taking it to the rheumatologist. You know what? Our pediatrician was spot-on. Even if it was a mild rheumatic issue (but I don't think it was), the course of treatment he suggested would have fixed the problem, and isn't that what matters most? Evan's pain was addressed, its source was identified, and the problem was solved. Though I could have brought it up with the rheumatologist (and been justified in doing so, given the boys' history), the pediatrician was the best choice for the first point of contact. He solved the problem, we didn't have to wait months to be seen, and we preserved the more "scarce" resource of the rheumatologist!

The Next Step

Of course, sometimes the pediatrician won't have the answer. A good one will tell you that and refer you to the right place. When Grant's pain

TACKLING PAIN AT HOME

In addition to regular medications, there are several things you can do at home to help alleviate some of your child's pain:

- warm baths
- heating pads
- ice packs
- alternating ice and heat to "confuse" nerves
- gentle massage
- encouraging light exercise
- distractions—television, movies, video and board games, phone calls and video chats with friends and family
- laughter
- sleep

levels were so high and we didn't know what to do, an exam by the pediatrician wasn't enough. He referred us to rheumatology for a follow-up. When rheumatology couldn't give us answers either (his labs were not correspondent with his pain levels), she referred us to a counselor.

Grant was not ready to add a new doctor to his long list of specialists, especially not a psychologist. If Grant wasn't onboard, I doubted that the whole process would be effective. We met in the middle and compromised on seeing the school social worker, with whom he already had an established relationship. A few sessions in, the school social worker told me he felt Grant had a good handle on his emotions, but the pain was bad enough that he believed Grant was suffering from burnout. We needed to rework some routines and rules so he could have a little more joy back in his life, but in his opinion, there was something more there than just psychological pain.

Armed with this new information, I approached the pediatrician again, who concurred that Grant's issues did not seem psychological, but agreed that he could see signs of burnout as well. It was time to do more (in both areas), and we were referred to the pain clinic.

Pain Clinics–Powerful Tools

Sometimes referred to as a pain management clinic (PMC), this is a healthcare facility devoted to alleviating chronic or acute pain. Like any other facility, it's important to do your research before deciding on which clinic is right for you and your child. The focus, staff, philosophy, and treatments can vary widely from one facility to the next. Depending on the particular clinic, you may see a different mix of specialists and therapists, but in most cases there will be psychologists, physical therapists, and complementary/alternative therapists.

Some people might view the pain clinic as a little hokey, on the edge of real medicine, but not quite a discipline in and of itself. Truthfully, I was a little skeptical, too. I thought "*What more could they do for him that the other specialists couldn't?*" Attitudes toward pain management, especially in pediatric cases, have undergone major transformations in the past 40 years, and these clinics are gaining more and more respect within the mainstream medical community. Pain clinics are being recognized more often as a separate discipline that focuses on the whole person and not just the pain.

At the time we were referred to the PMC, we were willing to try just about anything. Since Grant's case was complicated and he was taking so many medications, I didn't want to embark on any course of treatment that was not embraced by his current medical team, especially if some of the therapies involved thinking out of the box. He had already been through so much, and I wanted to find the right fit for him on the first try if at all possible, even if it meant traveling a distance to get there. After researching pediatric pain clinics all over the country, we decided that the highly acclaimed program at UCLA was the best fit for us (even though we lived halfway across the United States) and set about making arrangements to be seen.

While I recognize not everyone has the ability to pick up and travel cross-country for appointments, we felt strongly enough about this clinic to do whatever we could to make it work. I booked budget flights and planned in advance. The clinic's support staff was wonderful, squeezing us in so we could maximize the most appointments in the minimum number of days. The school sent us off with homework and even allowed Evan to come with us to participate in the sibling research study. In addition, I was fortunate enough to have extended family that lived near the clinic and who generously allowed us a place to stay, a car to drive, meals to eat, and a fridge to store meds whenever we needed it, giving us a real home away from home. In retrospect, this is one of the most important things we did for Grant and, later, for Evan as well.

Our first visit to Mattel Children's Hospital UCLA was packed full of visits from all types of specialists. True to what we had been told, Grant's case was considered by the entire medical team—each type of specialist that Grant had seen at our "home" hospital came *to him* at his first clinic visit. It was so refreshing! They each approached him as his own person, completed their exams, and asked for his input. We spent quite a bit of time with the doctors from the pain clinic and rheumatology and found the plan we used in Chicago was very similar to the treatment program they would use for him, but with a few additions and minor changes.

The folks at the pain clinic did not think his pain was "all in his head." Grant had suffered through a very intense and painful experience between the onset of JIA symptoms and the DRESS syndrome. He had experienced pain for such an extended period of time that they believed he had an "amplified pain syndrome," which occurs when the body experiences pain for so long the brain refuses to shut off the signals for intense discomfort, even when there is no longer appropriate stimulus.

As a result, Grant was prescribed a short course of medications to "reboot" his system, along with a number of complementary and alternative medicine (CAM) therapies to help soothe his parasympathetic nervous system. Although there were many CAM choices available, we allowed the doctor to choose which modalities she thought Grant would benefit from most and went from there.

The doctor also recognized that Grant's lack of sleep created additional problems that prevented him from getting better. Sleep loss can increase a child's perception of pain, making them irritable, moody, and unable to function properly—contributing to the vicious cycle of pain. By consulting with rheumatology, she was able to change one of his nighttime rheumatology meds to something that still reduced inflammation, but also helped him sleep better.

Another factor this doctor wanted to address was the way we had been handling Grant's pain. Although we had been doing a pretty good job, my attempts to accurately chronicle the cycles and intensity of his pain were inadvertently reminding him of the discomfort and causing him to focus on those feelings. Based on the doctor's suggestions, I no longer asked him how he was feeling, but started to make and record my own observations, only noting his responses when he offered them to me. He would still wake in the middle of the night and need my help to reduce the pain to a bearable level, but I would focus on the soothing, rather than the level of pain he was experiencing and why it was there.

In our case, the pain clinic was covered under our health insurance and so were a few of the CAM therapies, while others were out-of-pocket expenses. We did the first round of treatments with the therapists who worked through the UCLA program, who then provided us with information on how to find a reputable practitioner in our area. A few weeks later, after several visits with each, we returned to see the doctor.

The difference was nothing short of amazing. Although he was not yet back to the "normal" pain levels corresponding to the inflammation markers in his labs, Grant had improved significantly. He gave the doctor an honest assessment as to which modalities aided him the most (including acupuncture, which he agreed helped him a lot, but he liked the least) and which ones were less beneficial. He was sleeping better, and his mood and concentration had improved as well. The doctor adjusted his support

COMPLEMENTARY AND ALTERNATIVE THERAPIES

Pediatric pain clinics typically offer a variety of complementary and alternative therapies designed to reduce your child's discomfort, including:

- massage therapy
- craniosacral therapy
- music and/or art therapies
- hypnotherapy (psychotherapy using hypnosis)
- psychological counseling
- physical therapy
- acupuncture
- yoga (Iyengar)
- psychiatric counseling/psychotherapy
- nutrition/supplements/herbs
- meditation
- biofeedback

Note: Even when working through a PMC, be sure to gain the approval of your primary medical team before including any new therapies, medications, or supplements.

plan and gave us additional direction on things we could do to improve his progress. Within a few months, he was back to the appropriate levels of pain for the type of stimulus or inflammation occurring. We finally started seeing glimpses of the "old Grant" again, and he was able to return to school full time.

We continue to visit the doctors and therapists through the UCLA program every few months. The CAM team therapists see him each time we go there in order to track his progress, since so many of his treatments are done out of state, and they want accurate reports to bring back to his California team. Our visits have been spread further and further apart as Grant has continued to improve, and we have actually started looking forward to these trips.

Although the experience may be different for everyone depending on the doctors you see, the treatments prescribed, the therapists with whom you work, and the program you choose, deciding to visit a PMC can be a powerful tool in learning to control your child's pain. If you are unable to attend a pain clinic with your child, I highly recommend Dr. Lonnie Zeltzer's book *Conquering Your Child's Chronic Pain*, coauthored by Christina Blackett Schlank. Many of the tips and techniques we learned at the pain clinic are included in her book. It's not a substitute for a clinic visit, but it is an excellent resource for managing your child's pain.

When it comes to pain clinics, I am now a believer. If your child is experiencing excessive discomfort, I hope you will consider finding the right PMC for your family. Not only did it give my child a new lease on life, and a very welcome respite, but it taught Grant how to control his pain, rather than allow the pain to control him, which will be a valuable tool for his entire life.

PART TWO

Life
Goes On

Juvenile arthritis should only be a part of your child's life, not the central focus for them or you! "Winning the game" against JA means raising the healthiest child possible, mentally, emotionally, physically, and spiritually. Once the medical portion is on track with a diagnosis and treatment plan, it's time to start considering the rest of the picture, which is how to manage life with JA: how to live and even thrive, despite its presence.

When JA makes its entrance into your family's life, few things will be the same. This isn't always a bad thing, but it will be different. The key to being as happy and productive as possible is to anticipate the big changes and be ready for them.

There is an excellent essay by Emily Perl Kingsley entitled "Welcome to Holland." If you haven't read it before, you should. To summarize: If all your life you had planned a trip to Italy and you finally took that trip, but the plane landed in Holland instead, how would you feel? It wouldn't be the trip you always dreamed of, but it could still be a wonderful trip! Originally written for parents of children with special needs, it also applies in our case. Although our children may not be able to do some of the same things they used to, we can replace those things with other activities, which may be just as special. I wouldn't choose to spend a week in the hospital with my son, but when we have, it has brought us closer together. We usually have some pretty funny memories despite the setting. It's making the proverbial lemonade out of your lemons and teaching your children to do the same.

In the second part of this book, I hope to guide you through the rest of the process. Although the medical portion plays a huge role in learning to cope with JA, the illness is not just about the medical issues; there are so many more considerations to ensure the health and happiness of your whole child. Addressing these issues will help you make the most of your new normal, from working with your child's educators, and developing a support system, to keeping your own sanity.

CHAPTER EIGHT

Family Matters

From the moment you hear that your son or daughter has a serious or chronic illness, your thoughts immediately focus on your child. You wonder how this will affect his future, his life, his dreams, and, most of all, what you can do to help. What you don't think about, at least initially, is how much the diagnosis will affect everyone else. Although you may only have one family member afflicted with the disease (or in our case, two), you soon come to realize that it's really a family diagnosis.

No doubt about it, chronic illness affects the entire family. It changes the way you live, the way you feel, and the things you are able to do together. There is a definite division of "life before" and "life after" the diagnosis, which typically requires some major adjustments from all parties. The added stress can drive a wedge between family members, or bring them closer together. Sometimes it does both. Now, more than ever, it's important to maintain and foster relationships in both your immediate and extended family circles, which is a lot more challenging than it sounds. Nurturing these relationships will prove to be one of the most valuable investments of your time and energy that you make. Life goes on, in spite of the diagnosis, and ensuring your family maintains healthy relationships will help you avoid other potential problems in the long term.

Just the Two of Us

After our boys were born, I remember thinking it was tough to squeeze in "grown up" time with my husband. While immensely rewarding, the demands of raising children can make preserving your marriage a bit challenging. These hurdles are magnified when a chronic illness is added to the mix! Frustration, guilt, stress, displaced anger, and lack of time for each other can push couples apart. In many ways, having a chronically ill child is similar to having a newborn baby—requiring constant attention and creating thorough exhaustion—but with no end in sight. It can be very difficult (if not impossible) to make time for each other. In order for things to work, there must be an open line of communication and a willingness to try to appreciate what your partner is going through. The more honest and understanding you can be with one another about your *real* needs (not wants) the better your chances of not letting this diagnosis tear you apart.

Right about now, you may be expecting me to tell you how important it is to schedule an adult-only dinner or make time for a date night—that your relationship is a high enough priority that you need to make it happen. But I'm not going to do that. I'm not a marriage counselor or a psychologist (although I do have an almost ancient BA in psychology from our "before JA" days). More than anything, I'm a mom who has lived through a pretty traumatic time due to my son's chronic illness. I can tell you that in the middle of our crisis mode, there was *no way* a date night was being scheduled! Like having an infant, there were days that I was lucky if I had time enough to shower, eat a meal sitting down at a table (instead of in a car on the way to a clinic), or even sleep in the same bed as my husband (instead of holding vigil next to my son's bed).

Obviously, these are not the times to work harder at planning date nights. During serious flares or hospitalizations, you must focus on taking care of your child and doing whatever you can just to stay sane. I will tell you though, if you aren't careful, these are also the times that can drive you and your spouse apart.

You might be thinking, "What kind of advice is that?" I suppose it sounds a little cynical at first glance, but it's grounded in reality. The best way to survive these difficult days and stay connected is to:

- Understand what you're up against and keep each other informed.
- Make sure you and your spouse are on the same page (i.e., decide who will be in charge of what and what expectations are), which will help you get through a crisis with less resentment.
- Realize these intense times are probably temporary (and even in more serious cases than ours, can be cyclical, with *some* relief every now and again).

If date nights are out, and you are too utterly exhausted and wrapped up in the care of a different family member, what are you supposed to do to nurture your marriage? Communicate. Listen. Be patient and kind. Be honest about your feelings and clear the air before small grievances become big ones. And try to remember that little things can mean a lot at this stage of the game. For instance, when I knew my husband was coming home, starved from a rigorous practice, but there was no way I could take time to make dinner, I had his favorite take-out meal ordered, delivered, and waiting. Meanwhile, he would stop by the pharmacy for me on the way home and save me a trip out. Divide and conquer the things that need to be handled and absolutely cannot be ignored. Appreciate each other and look for the good. Don't take the small stuff for granted—a 30-minute snuggle or napping on the couch together before the next round of meds is due can be a way to stay connected. Remind each other that this too shall pass, and this crisis can't last forever. You can share your war stories later.

When things slow down or start to normalize again, *then* jump on the opportunity to reconnect and put effort into those classic marriage builders. Trying to be everything to everyone is not realistic, and it can create additional stress and resentment that can backfire on your relationship. It's better to be open, honest, and know *your* physical and emotional limits, so you can support each other. Instead of growing apart, you might just grow together.

What about Me?–Remembering the Healthy Sibling

Your spouse isn't the only one who may be feeling neglected. If you have other "healthy" children in the family, their sibling's chronic illness can be equally troubling for them. Healthy children crave your attention, too. They can often feel left out and hurt as most of your time and energy becomes focused on the child who is ill.

Since they are children, you may forget to provide them with age appropriate updates on their sibling's progress or condition. They may be frightened by the changes they see, and worry that the same thing will happen to them. Even though brothers and sisters may squabble, deep down they care about each other, and seeing a sibling in such a frail or painful condition can be traumatic.

There is a tendency to keep things from children as a way of protecting them. However, just because they're young, it doesn't mean their worries are any less stressful. It's important to be honest with your other child(ren) and available to address their questions and concerns. Recognizing their fears and offering reassurance can make them feel more secure.

It's also normal to see some aggression, jealously, or anger regarding the situation. Younger children may act out just to garner additional attention. Although I don't condone bad behavior, this is usually a good time to allow some extra latitude. In these circumstances, a meltdown might not warrant a quick punishment, but it should require a talk, a consequence, and an apology, with a warning that the next time a punishment will be enforced. Taking things a little easier also gives you a chance to handle the situation in a calmer way, as the additional stress that you will be facing could shorten anyone's fuse.

Just as with the "sick" child, trying to maintain as much normalcy as possible will help add stability to the "well" child's ever-changing life. Overcompensating will come back to bite you later, as you may end up with a monster on your hands, while undercompensating (thinking you can always make it up to them later) can result in deep-seated hurt and anger. It's all about balance.

My younger son took the first round of hospitalizations for his older brother quite well. I was staying with Grant around the clock at the hospital, while my husband was home with Evan, bringing him for after-school visits. As a result, I missed making the cupcakes I had promised for his class Valentine's Day party. Evan assured me it was no big deal—he had told his classmates how sick Grant was, that he was in the hospital, and we had no idea when he would be out. For a time, the attention he was missing from me was being made up by sympathetic teachers and friends. Evan missed us, and he was visibly worried, but he was also enjoying the consideration he was getting from outside the family, along with eating pizza for dinner, playing extra video games with his dad, and having more control over the TV remote.

However, after a few days, when "Evan's brother being in the hospital" was no longer big news at school, the reality started to set in. We were still living it, but Grant's hospitalization was old news to everyone else. The longer we stayed at the hospital, the more serious Evan realized things were. He missed talking to his brother after lights out, and he liked the lunches I packed better! Everything was turned upside down. Evan wasn't being kept in the loop (even though we weren't completely sure what was going on with Grant either), and we hadn't taken the time to figure out what was going on in *his* head. Evan was putting on a brave face, but what he was feeling on the inside was a completely different story.

To add insult to injury, earlier in the year I had volunteered to chaperone a field trip that was scheduled about a week after Grant was released from the hospital. My mother was helping out and was planning to stay home with Grant, while I spent a couple of hours with Evan and his class at the county courthouse. Two days before the field trip, we got some bad news: Grant's latest labs had come in and his liver numbers were alarming. He would have to be readmitted right away. When I hung up the phone, I turned to find Evan staring at me intently. With a quiver in his voice, he said, "But you will *not* ditch me on my field trip, right? They are counting on *two* moms, and you promised."

I didn't know what to say or do. Before Grant's illness, if you needed treats for the party or an extra hand to help out at school, I was your gal. I was the mom who always tucked my kids in and kissed them before bed, helped with their homework, and met them after school. I was very hands-on and I didn't play favorites, but over the past two weeks I had spent every waking moment with my older son. Meanwhile, my then 9-year-old had my *divided* attention for a grand total of three or four hours *combined*. I felt like a schmuck and a failure as a mom, a point that was driven home when Evan added, "And don't think Dad or Grandma can take your place either. Miss S likes it when *you* come to help."

You can probably guess how this played out: I missed the field trip. Possible liver failure, non-viral hepatitis, and a hospital admission for son number one trumped a visit to the courthouse with son number two. That doesn't mean I felt good about it though. Evan was starting to feel hurt, like a second-class family member. He even accused me of being only Grant's mom. It was like déjà vu—that's exactly what Grant said when Evan was born! On the other side, Grant not only felt bad physically, but also felt guilty that his illness was causing Evan to feel so left out. All of this family drama, *on top* of the true medical crisis, was a recipe for stress overload (and my husband and I weren't having any "dates" that week either!).

Fixing What's about to Be Broken

Although it would have been *very* easy to play ostrich and stick my head in the sand, waiting out the medical storm and then cleaning up the aftermath, I didn't. While "enjoying" some down time at the hospital, watching Grant nap, I contacted Evan's school. I let them know what was going on and arranged for him to meet with the staff social worker in my absence. I spoke with his teacher and worked out a flexible plan to do something else for Evan with his class, as soon as I could get a free day. Nothing was going to stop me from parenting *both* my children; I was just going to need a little more time and some extra help.

Truthfully, it was still a struggle. I hate to think how hard it would have been if I had not put these ideas into play right away. We were very lucky to have good neighbors and classmates who would give Evan a ride (and social time) to and from school, a very caring teacher, and a wonderful social worker who helped him work through his feelings, whether he felt like he needed to or not. But, of course, no one can replace a parent.

It still took time to figure out a balance for both kids that was practical under the circumstances, but I refused to give up. I allowed other people to help more than usual, and also encouraged Evan to participate in more visits to friends' houses, sleepovers, parties, etc. What I focused on most was making Evan feel special, since so much of the attention was targeted toward Grant. I made a point to spend one-on-one time with Evan once a week, *without* scheduling a firm day or time—I knew better than to set myself up for failure when Grant's health was still so volatile. Cancelling more activities with Evan due to an unanticipated trip to the doctor would only make him feel worse than he already did. Instead, I made sure that by the end of each week, I had done something special for him, and that we had spent some quality time together.

The same way I had allowed Grant some leeway with firm family rules also applied to Evan. If the only way I could manage to squeeze in our one-on-one time before the week was over was to let him stay up late with me one night, so be it. The younger brother is always thrilled when the older sibling has to go to bed earlier than they do! We would catch up on a favorite TV show we had recorded or watch a DVD. Occasionally, Evan got to pick the entire dinner menu for the evening and help me prepare it. I received permission to pick him up from school for lunch now and then. If I had an "easy" day with Grant, I could show up at the school and take him out for a slice of pizza and conversation, just the two of us. Also, the school approved of my allowing him one hooky day each term. He was able to choose the day, as long as there were no tests or special events/reports at school on the selected day. When Grant was able to go back to school, Evan used his days to plan an activity he would enjoy with me; something that Grant wouldn't necessarily want to do, like a visit to the soccer shop, a matinee movie of his choice, or lunch at a spot that only *he* really liked. Many days, Grant was too ill to go to school and Evan would resent that he was unable to stay home as well, so this was a perfect compromise (although Grant did complain that he never got to stay home "well" and have a fun day!).

The key to supporting the "other" child is being there for them as much as possible. It's different for every family and every circumstance. You may have to get creative with your ideas and solutions, but it's important to remember that JA affects *everyone* in the family, and those effects will have to be addressed in order to keep your *entire* family healthy and happy.

When It's Something More

When one child in the family suffers from a chronic illness, it's not unusual for the "well" child to act sick in order to regain their fair share of attention. This can be magnified with younger children, but even older ones may complain of headaches, stomachaches, or similar symptoms. Even if attention seeking is not the cause, the stress caused by the change in circumstances can lead to feelings of illness. For many siblings, worry that they might have the same illness can be overwhelming, and they can even talk themselves into symptoms. But what if it's something more?

Siblings of children with juvenile arthritis have a slightly higher chance of developing the same disease than others in the general population. It's important to keep an eye on them without driving yourself crazy or developing psychosomatic symptoms in them. Also, the well child could be developing something that needs medical attention in a completely different area, but being so focused on the sick child or signs of JA may cause you to overlook things you would normally pick up on.

In Evan's case, I was seeing quite a few complaints similar to Grant's in the early days before diagnosis. I started journaling his issues as well, but taking a cue from Dr. Zeltzer's book, I rarely asked him how things were; instead, I waited for him to tell me. I had learned that if pain was present, asking about it all the time could make it worse, by keeping it at the front of his consciousness. Even if it was "just for attention," asking him how he felt all the time just fueled the fire. If he felt bad enough, then I expected him to come and tell me. I tried to notice particular patterns, or the absence of any pattern. Was he lying in pain on the couch only until a friend called? Did he miraculously recover when it was time for his soccer game? I really didn't want to miss anything this time around, but by the same token, I didn't want to create a "mental" situation either. It was another tough balance.

I couldn't do it alone. As Evan's complaints escalated, I asked his teacher to keep an eye on him, too. Did she notice more stiffness in the morning or was he less involved with his friends? Did the school nurse see him more often, because he always had something wrong? His PE teacher was also a very valuable resource, able to review his activity level and exertion over time, along with any changes.

Teachers weren't the only helpers. Once again, our pediatrician came to the rescue. He was available to see Evan through all his injuries, whether serious, slight, or nonexistent. With a very active child involved in sports, it was difficult to know what was normal soreness, a hint of JA to come, or an actual injury. The pediatrician helped by being an objective third party and a trusted adult. Many times, I think Evan's visits to the pediatrician were more for his mental health than physical problems, but our pediatrician encouraged us to utilize him for that role. With his training, he was also able to help us keep an eye on any possible signs of JA without letting it take over our lives with worry. Knowing he was being followed by a medical professional allowed me to turn over some of that concern to someone else.

Sticks and Balls

Evan did end up being diagnosed with a mild case of JA. In the beginning, I watched him so closely to see if he had any of the signs we had seen with Grant, but what I learned is that two children, even with the same condition, can be affected very differently. In other words, JA can be as unique as the kids themselves!

In some ways, this is no different than any other aspect of childrearing. When I was pregnant with Evan, I thought I was ready. I had been pregnant before and had lived through the baby years once already. Both of my kids were going to be boys, and they were close enough together that I still had everything I needed—clothes, books, toys, you name it.

Grant loved balls. When he was only 7 months old, he would crawl around holding four to five balls at one time—one in each hand, one under his chin, and one or two in the space made between his knees by crossing his ankles! No toy was very interesting to him unless it had a ball somehow related to its use. When Evan came along, I had *all* the cool ball toys. But guess what? Evan wasn't interested. *He* liked sticks: baby baseball bats, giggle sticks, and wands of any kind. The closest thing to a ball that he favored was a round toy made up of—you guessed it— a bunch of sticks and beads on elastic bands. A ball made of sticks!

Grant was vocal, but Evan was not. None of Grant's clothes fit Evan, as they had completely different builds and were different sizes in different seasons. I soon realized that I didn't have things figured out after all.

A diagnosis of JA in your second child can be much like this story. You think you know this disease, and you do. You just may not know it in *this* kid. Remember that each case is different and suppress the urge to tell the doctor "but when _____ had that issue …" Each kid is an entirely different ball game. That doesn't mean your experience will go to waste. Some things will be just the same. You will still need to communicate with the doctors, handle the insurance issues, and maintain relationships with his school and the family. You will still need to journal and photo document changes in his or her health and symptoms and fulfill the challenging role of parent to a chronically ill child. Those things will be the same, and they will be easier the second time around. The hard thing will be to remember they are individuals, not just as people, but also within their illness.

A fellow JA mom with two affected kids told me once that it was sometimes easy to forget her second child was even sick compared to the first (who had a much more serious and complicated case), but looking at that same child next to other "well" kids put it all back in perspective. The second child was fighting a significant battle too, but it was overshadowed by a much more serious case in the family. As parents, we have to look at each child's case individually, and *not* in relation to their siblings, which can be difficult to remember.

Extended Family

I couldn't write a chapter on family matters without recognizing the importance of grandparents, aunts and uncles, cousins, and other extended family. From my experience, they can be the greatest source of comfort and help, or the biggest source of frustration and hurt. Like everything else in life, some family members "get it," and others do not, despite any attempt you make to educate them. As they say, we can pick our friends, but not our family; therefore, you may find you are dealing with a mixed bag of personalities and views on your child's illness.

If you are one of the lucky ones, you will have family members ready to step up and help wherever and whenever they can, and who don't question your child's medical treatment plan. My mom was an amazing help, staying with us and doing whatever we needed in order to facilitate the hardest times. My mother-in-law was also fantastic, with a standing offer to come across the country any time we needed her. Some family members kept in contact with the kids, with calls, cards, and goodies in the hospital, but others seemed to drop off the face of the earth. Some offered to help, but never made good on their offers.

Nearly all the other JA families I have talked to have had similar experiences. Some family members just don't know what to say or do, while others are too overwhelmed and can't face what is happening. Regardless of the reason, even though it's hurtful, you can't take it personally.

Another difficult aspect of dealing with family can be the unsolicited advice—"Hey, I saw this on *Dr. Oz* and your treatment plan is all wrong," or "No one else in the family has had this, so you're blowing it out of proportion, it's not that big of a deal," or "He looks great, so he must not be *really* sick anymore" or my personal favorite, "Relax, I know he's going to grow out of it." Admittedly, I haven't always bit my tongue. Sometimes I say that as soon as they earn their medical degree, I'll be sure to come to them for advice, but in the meantime, I'm sticking with the real doctors. But, for the most part, I try to smile, grit my teeth, and move on. These people are family, so they won't be going anywhere anytime soon. Better not to make the situation any worse.

I have tried to educate everyone (not just family) who comes into regular contact with my children on what they are going through so they can act accordingly. If my son is lying on the couch with a back flare, Grandpa should probably pick a different cousin to fetch something in the attic for him. However, despite your attempts to educate, some people just won't understand, and never will. Don't spin your wheels with them. Teach the other family members as much as you can, and hopefully after everyone else comes around and understands it, they will, too. You have enough things to worry about, so don't wear your heart on your sleeve or start world war three. That will only make things more difficult!

If there is absolutely no way of remaining civil or developing understanding, sometimes it's appropriate to put a little distance between family members until feelings are a little less fresh. One family member noted several times how "huge" Grant had gotten on steroids (within earshot of him no less), despite being warned in advance and told of his sensitivity. As you might guess, we became a little more careful about who we let into our inner circle for a while, both friends and family.

Even the most well-meaning family members can cause difficulties! Communication with these extended family members is important as well. You need to educate them on the disease, forewarn them of the changes (physical and emotional), and prepare them, especially if they haven't seen your child on a daily basis. Family should nurture your children during the hard times, not contribute to them, even inadvertently. You are the judge of what is best for your children, and sometimes that involves protecting them from family, as well.

THE OTHER KID by EVAN

Having your brother in the hospital isn't just hard for him; it's tough for the sibling, too. I know because my brother has been hospitalized several times. Even though I understood he was sick and I was worried about him, I sometimes felt unappreciated and that no one cared about me. Instead of always picking me up from school and asking about my day, my parents would sometimes make me walk home and not even pay attention to what happened to *me* that day. And, because they felt like they were slacking on behavior with the sick kid, it all came down on me—it seemed like they were always so harsh. Every little thing was a big problem. It's also hard when almost everyone you know is asking about your sibling without bothering to ask how you have been.

At times, I felt so bad that all I wanted to do was sit in my room all day. But, that's not the answer. There is a way to fix it! You can always find good friends or another adult to talk to and help distract you. It also helps to talk to someone about how much you're worrying about your sick sibling. My brother had a 50 percent chance of dying and that made me feel terrible. He was always the one who played with me, got me out of trouble, and persuaded my dad to let me play my favorite sport. When he was in the hospital, it almost felt like all that was going to come to an end. It was scary. To all you siblings out there, I know it's hard for you, too! Keep your head up and don't doubt yourself; just believe in yourself and you'll get through it.

Now, for parents who have a really sick kid and a "well" kid, I know it's hard, but you need to always acknowledge the other child because they might feel like they don't even have a family at the moment. When the sick sibling is feeling fine, try to spend some one-on-one time with the other kid, doing something he'll enjoy. Trust me, he or she will appreciate the effort! Yes, most of the time the sick child is feeling very bad and you feel like you should pay attention to him 24/7, but you shouldn't. You need to see if your other child is hurting. For instance, I had arthritis, too, but my parents thought I was faking and just trying to get attention at first. If your other child is complaining about pain, always check with your doctor or pediatrician. And kids, be honest with your parents so they can trust what you say and that won't happen to you!

Parents, you will get through this and it will make you braver and tougher. Like my mom, you will probably also feel like you are on your way to receiving a medical degree ☺. Even though dealing with this disease is really hard, you will keep going and spread the word to other people so if their kids have these problems it won't get too serious.

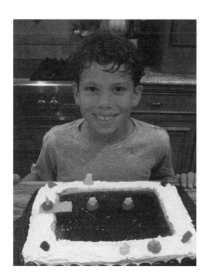

When my brother was ill, my mom and I made this cake. I picked it out of a cookbook and we went shopping for all the ingredients together. Even though it was over three years ago, I still remember making it because of the special one-on-one time with my mom—and I was really proud of the result!

CHAPTER NINE

Your Cheering Section

As you can imagine, I have attended quite a few sporting events in my lifetime. Even though the players and coaches are doing all the heavy lifting, I have learned to appreciate the importance of a cheering section. They can give you the boost you need when times get tough. In fact, the fan base can be so crucial to a team's success that in football there is even a name for it: the 12th man. While there are 11 players on the field, the 12th man refers to the fans in the crowd. Their cheers can motivate the team, and the noise they make can distract or disorient the opponent. Just as the fans' importance has earned them an honorary NFL position, your cheering section plays an important role on your team. They can keep you going when you and your child are just so tired of JA. They can motivate you to stay engaged in life outside the illness and provide support when you need it most. Having your own cheering section is like adding another player to your team.

Your cheering section can be made up of people from many different areas and may even overlap from another part of your "game." At times, the doctors have even taken a seat in our cheering section, pushing us to reach that next milestone and celebrating with us when we get there. In addition to family and friends, you might be surprised by where your biggest fans come from.

Family, Friends, and Strangers

Family can be very helpful, but keep in mind that family members may not always "get it." If they don't, it's important to educate as much as possible, since these are the people who will always be in your child's life. It's not wrong, however, to put a little distance between your immediate family and those who may be creating more stress. The best way to beef up this part of your cheering section is to enlist the help of a family member who *does* understand and is willing to help the others come around without creating additional stress for you.

Friends don't always have the same connection as family. Unfortunately, you may find that some just disappear when your child becomes ill. They could be worried about catching something, unable to handle the emotion, or unwilling to accept a new type of relationship. We had a couple of good friends (and at least one family member) who told us the situation was just too depressing for *them*, after we learned of Grant's JIA. Others become wrapped up in their own lives and don't have time for you when you are no longer participating in the same activities or when the diagnosis becomes old news. Although this is a relatively common occurrence, most JA families are still shocked when it happens to them.

On the bright side, there are always a few friends that step up to provide more help and support than you would have expected. Some of our former acquaintances have become very close friends since Grant's diagnosis. Going through this ordeal taught us who our real friends were and allowed us to create stronger, even lifelong bonds.

Strangers can also be a surprising source of support. Seriously! From the receptionist at the clinic to the phlebotomist at the lab, people you don't know personally, but who are familiar with your child's diagnosis, can make a positive impact. A kind word during a blood draw—"wow, you were the bravest kid this morning!"—or an inside joke with the receptionist who says "hope we *don't* see you next week" after a few unscheduled visits can give you that much needed boost on an off day. Other "strangers" such as hospital roommates, foundation employees, familiar families being seen in the same clinic, and even online friendships can be a very important part of your cheering section. At times, they can provide even more support than your friends and family, since they share a common experience and really understand what your family is going through.

KNOWING WHAT TO SAY

One of the topics that come up frequently among families coping with JA is the things people say. Just like the 12th man in football, some comments can be disruptive noise while others provide a true boost. Together with other JA families, I have compiled a helpful list of what to say and what not to say. You can share this list with your family go-between, a trusted friend, or even your child's educators to help them become a more effective cheering section.

Things NOT to Say

- **But (s)he doesn't *look* sick.** Autoimmune diseases under the JA umbrella operate on the inside. Their bodies are attacking themselves. Just because a child looks well doesn't mean he or she is well, or even feels well. Sadly, if these children "looked" sick, they may get a little more understanding and empathy.
- **At least it's not cancer.** No, but it can be a potentially fatal disease that few understand, and it receives far less research and funding dollars. Some forms of cancer can be cured. Arthritis can only go into remission. There is no cure.
- **Are you sure it's arthritis?** Well, yes. That's why we have been to the hospital/lab/doctor so frequently!

- **Thank goodness your other child is well.** True, for now? In the meantime, I worry every day that things will be the same for the other children in the family, and the non-affected child feels guilty for being well. It's not a trade-off. I feel horribly for my ill child, period. Other children being well doesn't change the way I feel about *his* struggle!

- **I'm sure he'll grow out of it.** Yes, I'm sure you are, because you haven't heard the prognosis straight from the doctors or researched this issue like I have. We can hope for remission, but he will *not* grow out of it, so please don't marginalize what he's going through.

- **Kids don't get arthritis, it's just growing pains.** JA is not the same arthritis you get from a sports injury or aging. It's not an "old people's" disease. It's an autoimmune condition that causes children's bodies to attack and damage themselves. It's very painful, and it's *not* just growing pains.

- **I could never give my child all that medication, who knows what it will do to him.** I don't like giving my child serious drugs with possibly dangerous side effects. I hate being the shot giver and administering medications that cause nausea, headaches, excessive weight gain, and increase cancer risks. However, I also hate leaving him untreated in pain with the possibility of permanent damage even more. Please don't rub it in. It's hard enough without your incredulity.

- **Why wouldn't you just use "_____"?** (Insert supplement, herb or food here.) **So many people have success with that.** Again,

I trust my medical team. I don't mind if you bring something to my attention, but don't assume it will cure my child or be angry if we don't rush to try it. Believe me, any non-drug therapy approved by our doctors that doesn't interfere with the researched and proven treatments, we are willing to give a shot. Chances are, we've tried (and even failed) using *X* months ago.

- **Isn't he "over" that by now?** No, it's a chronic illness. We hope for remission, but he will *never* be over it.

- **God doesn't give you more than you can handle.** Very true, but I don't think God would put this kind of suffering on a child either. Having JA isn't about God, although spirituality can be a comfort. Most families find this statement abrasive.

- **Are you sure he isn't faking/lazy/exaggerating?** Yes, I am. I have been with him at the doctor, I have seen the lab results, and I live with him. You don't even know the half of it. If you only knew how hard he pushed himself just to be told he ifaking/lazy/exaggerating, it would break your heart. Many times it has broken his.

- **You are so lucky to miss so much school. It must be nice to have that much vacation/free time.** Remember that the next time you are home sick with the flu, with all that free time! It's not fun. These kids miss their friends and want a normal life. Many families have to travel out-of-state to visit their rheumatologist. Seeing a city from inside a hospital or clinic is not a vacation, and missing school because you are too sick to go is not a break.

- **I know just how you feel.** Please don't say that unless you do.

You might be able to imagine, but unless you know us well or have it in your own family, probably not. These kids are courageous and put on a brave face to the world most of the time. Please do show them empathy, but don't patronize.

- **Why are you so serious? It's just a few aches and pains.** JA can damage organs and stunt growth. It can disfigure and cause blindness, as well as pain. It's far more than just aches and pains.

- **He looks great! So the meds worked and everything is fine now. Nothing to worry about, right?** Remember, there is no cure. If you knew how many medications we administer, all with their share of side effects, in order to keep him "looking so good" you would be shocked. We are grateful he is doing so much better, but there is also a price, so yes, we worry!

- **WOW. I hardly recognized him, he has changed so much.** Please don't draw attention to the things we know are happening. Steroids can cause acne and excessive weight gain. The chemo drugs can cause hair loss. Most kids are pretty conscious of the changes, and pointing them out makes them feel that much worse. We know you are shocked. We already saw it in your face. Please don't say anything and make it worse.

Things You Should Say

- **I can only imagine how hard this is for your family. What can I do to help?** Showing empathy, but not marginalizing what we're going through, means a lot. If you can sincerely offer to help, it means even more.

- **I'm not very familiar, can you tell me more?** We want to raise awareness for the chronic diseases under the JA umbrella! There are nearly 300,000 children diagnosed, but surprisingly few people really understand what it entails. Raising awareness will ultimately increase funding and improve the chances of finding better treatments or a cure. At a minimum, it will help you understand what we are going through!

- **I know he looks good, but how is he *really* doing?** This makes me feel like you care and you really "get it." Just because he is looking better doesn't mean things are easier yet. He could look horrible by the end of the day! The cycles with this disease can be pretty wild.

- **What a great kid. He is so amazing/happy/brave/strong though all this.** Thank you! These kids go through a great deal, and it's wonderful to be recognized and built up, especially when so much is at work against their self-esteem. It's true, too—these kids are amazing!

- **I know this is hard for all of you. You are doing a great job.** Parents need some affirmation, too. Sometimes it seems as though we are making gut-wrenching decisions for our kids on a daily basis. The right choice is not always clearly defined. It's nice to hear when you *do* think we've been doing a good job!

- **How are YOU?** It's very nice to be recognized for the things I'm going through in relation to my child's disease. I feel their pain, and so often I wish I could take it away from them. If I could, I would suffer through it instead of them. It's comforting to have a friend ask about *me* too.

- **I'm running by the grocery/pharmacy/coffee shop, can I grab something for you at the same time?** We will hardly ever ask, but if you offer, we may just take you up on that, especially if it's not out of your way! A routine errand for you could be an insurmountable obstacle for me today. Don't doubt the power of a small gesture.

- **Can I have one of your other kids over to play/pick them up from school while you are at the hospital/doctor?** Just knowing I have a few people who are willing to help and whom I can fall back on if I need to is a huge relief and a worry off my mind. If you say it though, please mean it.

- **I am thinking of you/praying for you.** If you mean it, this gesture is simple and comforting. It's nice to know we are not forgotten when we often drop off the face of the earth! Thoughts and prayers are always appreciated. This doesn't mean we have to break everything down about God's plan for us—just that we are included in your prayers.

And finally, the few last things on the "do" list aren't saying things at all. Just listen. Sometimes we need a friend to hear what we're going through, a shoulder to cry on, or someone to giggle with, without comparing our situation to someone else's or offering advice. Anticipating a need, like bringing over a coffee or having a home-cooked meal ready for the family when they get home from the hospital, can mean so much. Shoot me an e-mail, give me a call from time to time, and don't be frustrated with me when I have to cancel our plans at the last minute. I can guarantee I'm more disappointed (and needed the time out more) than you.

Sometimes, even when people mean well, it can be difficult to know what to say or do. Before I had a chronically ill child, I think I was guilty of all these faux pas at one time or another, and I'm sure you have been, too! When someone says something inappropriate, you can use the opportunity to educate. Try to remember that unless you've lived through something similar, it's almost impossible to comprehend the situation. Ignore the strangers who make you angry with their comments, try to enjoy the friendships you have, even if they don't always get it, and seek out new friendships with those who do!

Recruiting New Fans

It may seem odd to bring strangers into your trusted circle. Believe me, I understand! As a former NFL wife, I was very guarded about our private family life. It seemed counterintuitive to share details about ourselves with strangers online or offline. That is, until our first extended hospital stay. After spending 10 days in a small room with another critically ill JA (specifically JDM) child and his parents, I learned you could make very good friends rather quickly. In all fairness, days in the hospital are like dog years—one day is equivalent to about one week on the outside. You either pack in about 20 hours of conversation each day or stare at the walls. There really isn't much time for sleep, with medical personnel coming and going at all hours, not to mention the hours you stay up to monitor your child's condition. Within a very short period of time, you either hit it off with your roommates or you don't, but, more importantly, you share a very intense time in your lives. We joked that the experience is similar to Stockholm syndrome, a type of traumatic bonding made stronger from the shared "captive" hospital experience.

We met the Smiths during our first hospital stay. While we were fairly new to the diagnosis and just learning the ropes, the Smith family was on day nine of their hospital stay. We had been told that we were only staying overnight for observation. However, since the Smiths were seasoned visitors, they knew better: No one made it out of the rheumatology/oncology floor in a day. Anke Smith never contradicted the doctors, but she broke it to me gently that we might be staying for a bit. To be honest, I wasn't interested in getting too friendly (since we were only staying the night anyway), but little did I know that Anke would become one of my new best friends. She may have sugarcoated things a little, but she let me know how it was going to be, and she was spot-on every time—we ended up staying for 10 days.

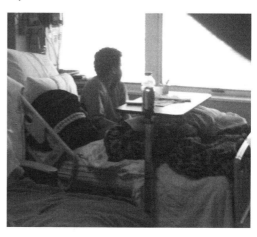

Grant's room during a hospital stay, including my "nest" with egg-crate-foam padded chair.

During our stay, Anke was the veteran training the rookie. She encouraged me to ask for an egg-crate pad for both my chair and my son's bed, so what little sleep we did get would be more comfortable and restful. Since she had been at the hospital awhile, she already knew the ins and outs. We took turns going to the vending machines. We listened to the doctors' reports for each other and filled in the blanks once they had gone. It's so valuable to have another adult present to ask if you heard something right or missed something after the doctor has gone. We staggered naps so that someone was always keeping an eye on *both* children's monitors, in case we needed to call in a nurse. We even suffered a round of isolation for infectious disease together (false alarm, but it's funny now thinking of all the folks coming and going in their special suits while we were trapped in the room just like our kids!). In short, we became battlefield buddies in our own version of war. We spent more time together in that week and a half than I spend with my "regular" friends in months, and she was going through exactly the same thing that I was.

Our relationship didn't end there. The Smiths lived out of state, so once they were released from the hospital, they needed to come back for follow-ups. We had already "lived" together, so we asked them to stay with us during their trips back to see the doctor. From there, the friendship grew and blossomed. We have since vacationed together and visited each other's homes just for fun. Who better to have adventures with than other families who have the same concerns and limitations as you? We bounce potential courses of treatment off each other when given choices by the doctors; after all, who else would know just as much, or understand the risks and benefits like another family in the same boat? Having shared experiences made it easier to connect, support each other, and create a very real friendship.

Many children's hospitals are moving to private rooms now, so you may not get the opportunity to bond with another family as we did. There are other ways to make those connections without staying in the same room, but they will probably develop a little slower.

Online Lifelines

Other than Anke, I felt a little lost. Our doctors were leaning on the idiopathic (that is, literally *unknown*) diagnosis pretty hard, since most of what Grant was experiencing was so atypical. I really wanted to put a name on his condition so I could find other parents who were going through the same thing. I knew he had spondyloarthropathy, but I had not found anyone with that diagnosis who had an experience anywhere near as intense as ours. With Anke away, I felt more alone than ever.

JM Moms and Caregivers, a private Facebook group, came to my rescue. Although Grant did not have juvenile myositis (JM), it does fall under the JA umbrella, and many of the treatments were the same for him as those children. Anke had been invited to the group and asked about adding me. They welcomed me with open arms and the rest is history. As I began conversing with members of this online community, I realized the struggles with which we were dealing, both medical *and* personal, were the same. Someone from the group had always made it through to the other side and had good advice to offer. Questions asked on the message boards were typically answered hours or even days before the doctor could get back with us, often with the identical answer. Although I never took the postings as medical advice, 99 percent of the time these in-the-know parents provided me with answers that allowed me to better prepare for the time I *did* have with the doctor. I could say, "*I know several children taking X—is Grant a candidate, and if so, how should I anticipate handling the side effects?*"

Knowing others' experiences beforehand helped me ask better questions and get better care. When Grant was prescribed methotrexate (a chemo drug), I asked about the potential side effect of excessive nausea. I was told that normally they wait and see, but some kids did experience very severe symptoms while it barely bothered others. I insisted on being prepared for the worst, so the doctor gave us a prescription for a strong anti-nausea drug, just in case. Knowing this had been the circumstance for several kids on the JM board made me push for the prescription. Good thing I did, because Grant was one of the few kids who experienced significant side effects for the first 24–48 hours after his weekly injection. Eventually the doctor would have given us the prescription given his reaction, but being armed with the knowledge of *real* experiences from others helped me avoid an even more unpleasant experience for my child the first time around.

As I spent additional time on the boards, I learned more and more, and slowly I began to feel less crazy. Eventually, I was added to other online groups that related to Grant's many conditions. These folks became my lifeline, even though we had never met in person. While much of the discussion was medically related, over time the conversations became more meaningful. In the beginning, I kept my posts short and to the point, discussing symptoms, doctors, and even a few frustrations. As time went on, things became more personal, as other parents would check in on my child or follow our case. The boards weren't just question-and-answer bulletins, they were a community. In time, I got to know many of these families and developed very real friendships, despite the fact they were "online."

Shared experiences are a powerful connection. Postings led to friend requests, private messages, and even phone calls. Some we have since met in person, others are so far across the country or the globe that we have not yet had the pleasure, but each one of these online friends has been valuable in their own way. We have also formed a few friendships like this from clinic visits, but truthfully, there is not enough face-to-face time to really develop a relationship. In most cases, the seeds of these friendships were sowed after meeting many times in the clinic waiting room, but grew through Facebook, Twitter, Instagram, texts, phone calls, and e-mails.

Connections for Kids

While these relationships are great for us parents, the kids need friends who really understand them and can be part of their cheering section, as well. Like adults, your child's "normal" friends may not "get it" either. It can be difficult for a child to comprehend how their friend could be a great athlete in the ball game on Saturday, but then be too sick to play with them after school on Monday. Having friends who share the same experiences and can empathize is important for your child's well-being, even if they don't recognize the need.

About a year into Grant's diagnosis, after we started going to the pain clinic at UCLA, Grant became involved in a peer study. The theory was that matching children with others like them (as well as some who were getting better and others who were worse) would help them cope with the issues they were facing in relationship to their illnesses. This particular study focused on pain, so not all the children had the same condition, but many of them were rheumatology patients. The families involved were spread all over the country, so the sessions were conducted over the telephone. The calls were for children only, except for a licensed health professional who would listen in and only intervene if the conversations were moving in a negative direction.

These sessions really opened my eyes. Grant had been getting more and more depressed, feeling like there was no end in sight and that no one really understood how he felt. After he started the study, things changed dramatically. When he spoke to the kids who had it worse, he started to appreciate where he was in his journey and feel grateful. At the same time, he was able to give those same kids hope that soon they might get to the same level as he was. When Grant had sessions with kids who were experiencing nearly the same things as he was, it allowed him to relax, commiserate, and validate the feelings he was having. It meant a lot to find other kids who knew exactly what he was going through.

The last group of kids included those who were doing better than he was, including those in remission. Talking with these children gave Grant renewed hope that it could happen to him, too. I noticed a significant positive change in his attitude and coping skills over the few months the study was being conducted. Even though the friends from his "old life" were great and still a big part of his life, I knew we would need to continue to foster friendships that related to his "new life" as well.

Just like me, Grant has valued friends he has never met. Noah's mom, Lori (see "Sharing This Journey"), is one of my online friends (we met on a Facebook rheumatology parents' page) with whom I also text, e-mail, and talk with over the phone. Our sons have some of the same overlapping conditions, are the same age, and are both very athletic boys. Although we have never met in person, our sons support each other through frequent texts. They understand each other in a way that no other adult or "well" friend can. One of these days, we hope to get together in person when we are in the same part of the country. Despite the lack of face-to-face contact, the online friendships we have created are very valuable and very real.

SHARING THIS JOURNEY by LORI

Once you've received a diagnosis and developed a treatment plan, you can begin to deal with the reality that juvenile arthritis is part of your life. The emotional roller coaster may never really end, but you eventually get used to the ride and learn to handle the twists and turns this disease can take you through. For my 13-year-old son, Noah, the emotional roller-coaster included a good deal of anger and frustration. He has asked "Why me, God?" and proclaimed "It's not fair" many times since his diagnosis, and, to be honest, my husband and I have shared those sentiments. These feelings are normal for any child or parent experiencing a chronic illness, but you can't let them consume you. Managing these emotions is an important part of moving forward.

I'll admit that, in the beginning, I let my fears and frustrations get the better of me. In an attempt to "fix" my son, I tried to micromanage his diet. The doctors had told us that Noah was anemic, so it made sense that perhaps there was a dietary component to Noah's disease, and I thought I was doing something wrong. In addition to boosting iron, I began researching foods that increase or decrease inflammation in the body. I went down every avenue I could find trying to change his eating habits. Of course, trying to change the eating habits of a 13-year-old boy is not easy, not to mention the difficulty of sorting through the huge volume of available information. Can we say *more stress*? I decided I needed help.

While searching for a support group on Facebook, I came upon a band of women who had children with JA. This special group of moms was truly a godsend. Though they were spread across the country and from different walks of life, they were joined by a common bond—and they could relate to every emotion I was experiencing. I could turn to these women with my questions or if I simply needed to vent. They offered advice, support, and even diet recommendations. Through every step of our journey with JA, these ladies have been an invaluable resource. Now I know that seeking medical advice is always the first line of defense, but these women sure place a close second!

When I was contemplating a particular biologic and its side effects, I reached out to this group. One mom took time out of her day to call me and try to alleviate my concerns about giving my son this drug. Her words eased my mind tremendously, and she addressed my questions and concerns. Again, she did not replace the knowledge and advice of our doctor, but since she was a nurse who had done considerable research on these medications, she was a valuable source of information. More importantly, she was a JA mom, like me, who understood my apprehensions. Thanks to her advice, I was able to follow the doctor's recommendation with confidence.

That call came at just the right time. When Noah received his first dose of this biologic, he had a local reaction and his leg swelled around the injection site. The doctor recommended an antihistamine and told me not to worry—the swelling should subside in a few days. I posted our experience on the Facebook page, and within minutes, many moms responded with comments about similar occurrences and advice for what to do next time. Luckily, Noah didn't have another reaction like that again, but the support I received was beyond comforting.

There have been many other examples of this type of online support. I remember one day, in particular, I posted my concerns over Noah's feeling that he was the only boy who suffered from JA. Of course, he was not the only child to feel this way, which was confirmed by a number of other women on the site. One mom offered to have her son, who was the same age as Noah, text him. The boys connected and soon discovered they shared the same love of sports as well as their JA. To this day, the boys still periodically text, even though they live on opposite sides of the country. We hope to meet up with this family one day soon so our sons finally can talk in person. But even though they've never conversed face-to-face, their connection has helped my son tremendously.

In addition to online support, we have attended the local family education day sponsored by the Arthritis Foundation. It provided an opportunity to meet with different doctors and ask questions about JA. There were workshops available on a variety of topics, such as nutrition and physical therapy. While very informative, the social connections were equally valuable. Noah met several boys and girls his age who suffered with JA, and parents were able to meet and talk over lunch. We also learned about summer camps where Noah will have the opportunity to interact with and get to know other teenagers with JA, while having some fun.

In short, don't underestimate the value of making connections within the JA community, whether it's online, at conferences, camps, or other venues. Talking with others who understand what you're going through can be a form of much-needed therapy. I also believe that each story we share has the power to help another family. It's very comforting to know there are caring, compassionate people who are willing to help each other—and who are traveling the same path you are now walking.

Conferences, Camps, and Other Events

Meeting people online is not the only way to foster relationships with similar families and children. Most local chapters of the Arthritis Foundation offer free or low-cost events for families to connect. We have even attended a few out of our home district (while visiting grandmas in other states) and met some of our online friends in person!

Beyond family events, there are also conferences and camps to consider. Each year the Arthritis Foundation hosts an annual conference for juvenile arthritis in a different part of the United States. The conference is an excellent opportunity to learn more about JA, including new developments, along with meeting other families. There are also a number of camps specifically tailored to children with rheumatic diseases. Many local chapters of the Arthritis Foundation offer camps in the United States, and *Serious Fun*, founded by Paul Newman, offers 30 camps around the globe for children with serious illnesses. The wonderful thing about these camps is they allow the kids to be kids and reach past their illnesses to just have fun. Since the camps are focused on children with their specific problems, parents and children can be confident of their healthcare and safety while at camp, so they can be free to just "be."

Everyone needs a cheerleader now and then, especially when you're dealing with a chronic illness. When you get your cheering section in place, I think you'll find that dealing with your child's condition is much easier to handle than it was initially. Things will still be hard, but you won't be doing it alone, and that makes a big difference.

STANDING PROUD AND TALL by AMY

One month after her eighth birthday, my daughter, Kylie, complained of pain in her left foot. She was participating in the play *Annie*, which involved rehearsals three nights a week consisting of vigorous dance routines and a lot of standing. I chalked up her pain to all that activity and chastised myself for buying discount dance shoes.

Within several days of her first complaint, the pain became unbearable and Kylie was unable to walk on her foot. The area around her ankle was swollen, hot, and red. We went to the emergency room only to find there was nothing remarkable on the X-ray. But the pain got worse—soon Kylie was crying and begging me to help her.

I took Kylie to a podiatrist who suspected a possible shift in the growth plate and placed her in a cast for six weeks. Meanwhile, her right ankle began to hurt. She finally ended up in a wheelchair. (Kylie will tell people that one good thing that came out of it was meeting the actor John Stamos, who was performing in *Bye Bye Birdie* on Broadway. We got to go backstage and meet him, where he autographed Kylie's cast!)

When the cast came off in January, Kylie's pain was still severe and the podiatrist was mystified. By this point, she had missed 10 days of school in only two months. In early February, we went to the pediatrician who immediately ordered blood work. Two days later, I received a phone call at work notifying me that my daughter's sed rate was 39 (normal sed rate for a child is 15). She was also ANA positive, indicating a rheumatologic issue. Sadly, the doctor felt strongly that my little girl was suffering from some type of rheumatologic autoimmune disease. He gave me the name and number of a pediatric rheumatologist and told me to make an appointment.

On April 12, 2010, four and a half months after Kylie's chronic pain and inflammation had begun we were finally able to see the specialist. At this point, Kylie had pain in her knees and neck, as well. After reviewing the blood work and performing a thorough exam, she confirmed the diagnosis—polyarticular juvenile idiopathic arthritis. Hearing those words come from Dr. E.'s mouth solidified my fear.

"Where do we go from here?" I asked. We were given two options: joint injections or chemotherapy. *Wait, did you just say chemo*? I had always thought chemo was only used to treat cancer patients, so I was shocked to learn it's also a treatment option for JA. Initially, I was very reluctant to give my daughter chemo, so we opted for joint injections.

In May, we drove to the hospital where my brave little Button received corticosteroid injections in both ankles while completely awake. No anesthesia for this courageous girl! Kylie is very proud of this story: the doctor told us that the week prior an 18-year-old boy had come in for the same procedure, saw the needle, and said, "Don't do it! I want to come back and do it under anesthesia!" So Kylie loves to brag that she is braver than a grown man!

During that first summer, it was evident that Kylie's JIA was not only here to stay, but also spreading rapidly to other joints, including her knees, wrists, neck, and shoulders. She flared so badly that she was not able to enjoy any of the activities she usually does, such as swimming, running with her cousins, and doing karate. By August she started on methotrexate injections—the chemo drug I was so reluctant to use just a few months earlier. We quickly learned that methotrexate was indeed chemotherapy, which suppresses the immune system. If Kylie was exposed to a cold, she ended up with bronchitis. In fact, over the winter, she suffered through bronchitis, two sinus infections, an ear infection, and a nasty stomach virus. The catch is, when a child who is on methotrexate gets sick, she must stop the medication, allowing JIA to rear its ugly head even more, which means additional sick days. Yet, despite missing 21 days of school, Kylie was one of only three students in the fourth grade to earn the Presidential Award for Academics, having earned highest scores on state and standardized tests.

Even with these treatments, our next visit revealed there was still active arthritis in Kylie's ankles. By now, her ankles had experienced active arthritis for a year and a half and the doctor was concerned about permanent joint damage. She started to mention biologics or TNF inhibitors. Biologics are much newer than methotrexate, and therefore the long-term effects are unknown. To be honest, they scared me. But, I was also terrified of permanent joint damage, so we agreed to give them a try.

We discovered that the biologic burned intensely when injected. It's a terrible feeling to have to inject your young child with potentially dangerous drugs as it is, but when that medication stings so much she cries in pain, you can imagine how that feels. Despite the burn, Kylie endured these injections for 16 months before the drug began making her very sick. Many children have great success, but JA is one of those diseases where it's different for everyone. Now we are trying to figure out what the best treatment plan will be. While Kylie is happy to forgo the injections, it's frustrating to see her suffer from JIA and feel stagnant in her treatment.

But Kylie remains positive. Now a sixth grader, she stands proud and tall when someone inquires about her JIA. She looks them square in the eye and tells it like it is. I am beyond proud of my little girl. Recently, one of her teachers asked if anyone knew what arthritis is, and Kylie explained to her class all about JIA. They asked her questions and she answered them. She explained that childhood arthritis is different from adult arthritis and there is no cure. She explained that she gets two injections to try to combat the symptoms of JIA. Kylie and I believe it's important to educate others and spread awareness for the need of JA research, which is why we are proud advocates for the Arthritis Foundation (AF).

Throughout this ordeal, we have been blessed to attend three Juvenile Arthritis Conferences all over the country and hope to attend more. To be perfectly honest, I don't know where Kylie and I would be today without the JA Conference. Our first one became what I refer to as our social journey. It opened up a network of friends going through exactly what we're going through! To say the conference has been an invaluable experience would be a huge understatement.

The AF has also been a marvelous resource. Last year, they helped set up a meeting for Kylie and another girl with JIA to meet Byron Janis (a famous classical pianist who suffers from psoriatic arthritis). Truly enthralled by Mr. Janis' life story, Kylie said, "Mommy, I want to be just like him when I grow up." He inspired her to continue taking piano lessons, and even taught her a few tips for playing the piano when arthritis is attacking your fingers or wrists. At one point, Mr. Janis asked Kylie, "Do you ever think, '*Why me?*' about your arthritis?" Kylie's response is one I will never forget. She replied, "No. I think God knew I could handle JIA and He wanted me to help other children who are going through what I'm going through." How can that not make you smile?!

The next weekend was our first Arthritis Walk. We created a power team called Kylie's Kickers and proudly raised more than $3,000 for the AF. Kylie created T-shirts that said, "Kylie's Kickers. Let's Kick Juvenile Arthritis! Arthritis doesn't stop me!" She won a prize for the best T-shirt at the walk. We were also able to talk with AF members and reflect on the time since Kylie's diagnosis. I am so grateful to these folks for their support, as well as all they have taught me.

We also attended JA Day at the Nationals baseball game in Washington, D.C., where Kylie and I had the incredible experience of help-ing AF members pass out Kids Get Arthritis Too (KGAT) bracelets. While most people accepted the bracelets and put them on, they didn't want to know more about JIA. Some tossed them aside or refused to take one. But a few others stopped to ask us what juvenile arthritis was. I was shocked at how easily the words came to me as I explained that JIA is often an invisible disease—people are constantly saying, "But she doesn't *look* sick." Many were shocked to learn that these kids are on chemotherapy, which, in addition to suppressing the immune system, can cause moodiness, affected liver enzymes, headaches, hair loss, stomach upset/nausea, and other problems. Biologics also suppress the immune system and come with an increased risk of infection and lymphoma. Despite these scary side effects, we give our kids these drugs because there is currently no alternative. We know children who have endured joint replacement surgeries, deformities, and other serious problems due to untreated JIA.

The bottom line is that juvenile arthritis is not acceptable. No child should have to suffer like this.

CHAPTER TEN

Back to School

Education is arguably one of the most significant components in a school-aged child's life. In addition to the acquisition of knowledge, going to school has a social aspect that is also very important to a child's growth and development. However, attending school with any form of JA can be a challenge, and the plausibility of regular attendance can vary from case to case, or even across different time periods within the same case.

As in so many other aspects of our children's lives, parents are ultimately responsible for determining when it's right to send their child to school and when they should absolutely stay home. Unlike having a "simple" case of the flu, there are many other considerations to take into account besides fever or vomiting! The normal rules dictating when to send your child to school or when to keep him home don't necessarily apply to the child with JA. In order to make the best possible decision, it's important to work with both your child's doctors *and* educators to determine the best course of action.

All three perspectives (from the parent, the educator, and the physician) share a mutual goal: to include the child in as many normal, day-to-day activities as possible, including regular school attendance. Regular attendance will keep the child from falling behind academically (thus adding to the laundry list of problems they already have to face), as well as serve as a distraction from the difficulties they are currently facing. In fact, being too lenient regarding how often and when a child stays home can actually *increase* some problematic behavior, including focusing on pain, amplifying the feelings of helplessness, and reducing the amount of exercise and movement necessary to keep the child mobile. On the other hand, there are times when pushing a child too hard to attend as much school as possible can backfire. Resentment can build between a parent and child when the student really does *not* feel well enough to manage the day, yet the parent forces them anyway. Also, if a contagious illness is making the rounds through the school or the classroom, it may be more prudent to ride out the duration at home. Many JA children take immunosuppressive drugs that can make minor illnesses for others a much bigger issue for them. As I have stated before, the key is to find the right balance for your child.

Of course, that's not always as easy as it sounds. If you let your child stay home too often, you may be enabling him or her to be sicker than they are, thwarting their physical, emotional, and academic progress. If you push too hard, you can develop a rift in your relationship, expose them unnecessarily to additional illness, and fatigue them to the point of exhaustion, which may even make them more ill. So, where do you draw the line?

First and foremost, you must consider doctor's orders. If the doctor nixes the idea of school, it's because he or she perceives a real threat to the child's physical well-being. In my experience, if the doctor says "no," it's better to err on the side of caution, keep your child home, and then reevaluate the situation as time progresses. If the doctor encourages your child to return to school, stating there is no medical reason to keep him or her home, then you should progress to the next stage of evaluation. This doesn't necessarily mean the child is ready to attend full time though, as we learned from experience!

Consider ALL Perspectives

Shortly after Grant was released from his second hospitalization in a month, we got the green light from our team of specialists to send him back to school, with the warning that if any widespread virus started to make the rounds, we should probably keep him home for a few days. But Grant, normally a good student who enjoyed school, told us he didn't feel well enough and was not ready to go back to school. My husband and I didn't want him to fall behind in his studies any further or for him to use his illness as a crutch. If the doctor said he should go, then he should, end of story.

We were wrong. Knowing my child, I should have taken his words more seriously. Grant wasn't the type to take advantage of a situation, and he was always one tough cookie. If he said he wasn't ready, I should have trusted him more. Even though the doctors said he should go back to school, my son knew he shouldn't. He was still having episodic fevers from the arthritis, significant skin rashes and hives from the drug reaction, and was generally uncomfortable. In fact, sending him to school was fairly useless as the drugs he needed to take kept him dopey, which coupled with his discomfort affected his ability to concentrate. After just half days at school, he would come home exhausted and unable to do anything but sleep. He woke up stiff and in pain every morning. He was upset with me for not listening. It was miserable, but I was sure I was doing the "right" thing.

After about a week of this very difficult time for all of us, the wonderful teachers and administrators at Grant's school approached me. While they appreciated our commitment to getting him back in the classroom, they didn't feel that school was the right place for him at that particular time. Think about it: Your child's teacher spends more waking hours with him or her during the week than you do, which means they are a valuable resource when it comes to insight about your child. We were very lucky that Grant's teacher and principal knew him before he was ill and had a good handle on who he was and of what he was capable. Just a few days after I had forced Grant to keep going to school, they let me know that it was not the right decision, at least not yet.

Grant's attendance was just an exercise in tolerance, as far as they could see. He was there, but wasn't learning effectively, and they worried the exhaustion he was facing might even affect his ability to heal in the long run. This didn't mean they wanted to send him home just to make things easy; they truly wanted what was best for my son and had a plan to make things better for all of us.

This part of my story isn't meant to illustrate how the doctor isn't always right; it's meant to show that the medical component is only *one* part of the equation. Your child is more than a walking manifestation of a disease. There were many essential factors to consider in determining whether Grant was ready to attend school, and only one of them was the medical portion. Although Grant was technically healthy enough to attend school, his educators realized he was not ready or able to undertake the task of learning in a traditional environment yet. This was *their* area of expertise. His physical discomfort and drug-induced brain fog kept his teachers from being able to effectively do their job in the conventional manner. He wasn't able to *learn* under the circumstances, which is a huge factor when deciding if a child should go back to school. If he wasn't learning, then the primary reason for his attendance became null and void.

Another factor that should have been considered was Grant's feelings. He knew he wasn't ready and felt I just didn't trust him. Every child is different, but Grant had always been dependable and never tried to get out of going to school unless it was really necessary. This time was no different! For children who are a little less reliable in that area, I would encourage parents to put themselves in their situation. Given the circumstances of that particular day, if you had the same symptoms, could you effectively do *your* job at work? If you can't at least say a begrudging "sort of," then you may need to keep your child home.

Let the Plan Evolve

In the beginning, I was also confused by the randomness of this disease. How could he feel well enough to go to school today, but not yesterday or tomorrow? JA has no rhyme or reason. Today may be fine, but there is no guarantee for tomorrow or next week. We learned to evaluate each day independently. Working with the doctor, the educators, *and* my child, we were able to figure out what worked best for him and devise the right plan to keep him on track.

Just as JA has morphed and changed over time in Grant's case, so has his educational plan. In the early days, we found that the homebound program through our local public school was the best fit. Grant tired easily, and he qualified for a teacher to come to our home and work with him for a couple hours each day. Under the circumstances, this arrangement was perfect, as he was not very mobile and could only tolerate a few hours of concentration daily. One-on-one tutoring was very efficient, maximizing what little time he had between his illness and many doctor appointments with focused individualized instruction. It also helped to make his transition back into school a little easier, as his instruction stayed on course with the rest of his classmates.

After several months of homebound schooling and significant improvements in his health, we decided to try a modified school day, as Grant was also missing the social interaction with his peers. He was still eligible (and utilized) homebound services if the situation dictated, but we worked on gradually easing him back into a manageable program that included more school attendance.

We were very fortunate to be dealing with a school system that wanted to work with us. As is often the case with JA, Grant would take one step forward just to find that he had taken two steps back. As his situation changed, the school adapted, allowing him to do modified work, having a teacher come back to our home on a temporary basis, or even just going to school for lunch or social time if that's all he could do. Having an entire system of people there to support our son and help him attain his educational goals was very comforting to us as parents, as well as to Grant. Allowing him to come to school for limited times also helped him to stay connected to kids his age and did wonders for his mental health.

The school became another part of our "cheering section," but also a place where he could just be himself, focus on learning and friendships, and forget about disease and illness for a few hours a day. The teachers, administrators, and school nurse became part of our "dream team," helping to keep an eye on him and recognizing changes in his physical condition and/or mental attitude. Having this fresh set of eyes to observe Grant allowed us to assess how he was *really* doing. Also, attending school gave us a much needed break from each other (we had been spending 24/7 together for months). Going back to school, in *any* form, made the overall situation better.

Working with Your School

Ideally, this is the way things should work—schools and parents working together, being flexible and accommodating the needs of all students. Of course, it doesn't always happen this way. We were very fortunate to have an administration that was familiar with autoimmune diseases and their potential to make children look well when they are, in fact, very sick. We had a caring staff and great teachers who knew us before all the drama unfolded. Not everyone is this lucky.

If you are fighting an uphill battle with your child's school, it's even more important to get certain documentation and procedures in place. Having a specific plan will help your child benefit from school, rather than it being a point of stress and difficulty. Even if you have an amazing group of educators with whom to work, there are some suggestions and tools that can make the process go a little smoother for everyone, especially if the staff is unfamiliar with the challenges your child may be facing.

One of the most important keys to success in working with your child's school is maintaining an open line of communication. After diagnosis, it's a good idea to schedule a meeting with pivotal staff, administrators, and teachers who interact with your child on a daily basis, as well as those who are responsible for crucial decisions regarding your child at school. Many times, these folks are unfamiliar with juvenile arthritis and are unaware of what your child is dealing with or could face in the future. This is your opportunity to educate the educators.

The same techniques that work for communicating with the medical community also apply here. Be well prepared and thorough, but as brief as possible. Bringing handouts, such as a letter from the doctor, and printed information about juvenile arthritis can be helpful and serve as future references. Find out what type of communication they prefer: Does the school nurse prefer a phone call while teachers favor e-mail? Do administrators want to be copied on all e-mails regarding absences? If so, make sure to keep them in the loop when there are changes in your child's case. Accepting and recognizing this part of your team as valuable contributors to your child's overall well-being is a great place to start.

After the initial meeting, you may need to conference with certain teachers individually or even meet with the school social worker. It may take a while to get everyone up to speed and work out all the kinks, but it's time well spent. If there are problems with the plan or a particular staff member, it's best to address these issues as early as possible, before they take on a life of their own.

One of the best ways to avoid this possibility is to develop a concrete plan of action. Outlining the responsibilities of each party and stating the necessary modifications and considerations that may be needed eliminate the guesswork when it comes to caring for your child in the classroom. The most common plans used in the educational setting are the individualized education plan (IEP) and the 504.

The Importance of 504s and IEPs

Both 504 plans and IEPs are designed to offer protection to children with disabilities, but the content, scope, and purpose of each plan are somewhat different. A 504 plan refers back to section 504 of the Rehabilitation Act, which was passed in 1973 and states, "*No otherwise qualified individual with a disability in the United States, as defined in section 7(20) shall, solely by reason of her or his disability, be excluded from the participation in, be denied the benefits of, or be subjected to discrimination under any program or activity receiving Federal financial assistance or under any program or activity conducted by any Executive agency or by the United States Postal Service.*" This, of course, includes participation in the public school system. It's important to note that 504 compliance is *NOT* mandatory for private schools, unless they receive some type of federal funding.

The purpose of a 504 plan is to break down the barriers that prevent anyone with a disability from obtaining *equal* access to educational services. In order to be considered disabled under the Americans with Disabilities Act (ADA), there must be some type of impairment that limits one or more major life activities that an average person can perform with little or no difficulty, such as walking, sitting, sleeping, standing, reading, or learning, just to name a few. There are no age limits to the 504 plan. The directives created for your child's 504 can vary from other children's plans, based on their individual needs and the needs that are *identified* by the staff members who create it.

Speaking with other parents who have already developed a 504 plan for their child with a similar condition can be helpful, since administrators may not be aware of all the possible barriers to education that exist with JA. It's better not to reinvent the wheel! Parents who have already experienced the ups and downs of JA can provide valuable insight as to what services or accommodations may need to be provided as things change in your child's case.

The Individualized Education Plan (IEP) is covered under the Individuals with Disabilities Education Act (IDEA), which also includes special education and behavioral plans, in addition to any physical disability allowances (if there are any). The IEP covers students between the ages of 3 and 21 years and provides *supplemental* services, free of charge, that will allow them to progress in their general education. Parents are also allowed to request independent evaluation and must receive written notice if any changes are made to their child's IEP.

Deciding which plan is the best choice for your child will depend on his or her unique set of circumstances and is best chosen through collaboration between the school, family, and medical care providers. If there is considerable difficulty reaching a good balance or agreeing on an appropriate plan, it may be worthwhile to contact and retain an educational consultant—an independent professional who provides assistance in the facilitation of the development, approval, and execution of these types of plans. (See the Resources section on where to find samples of a 504 and an IEP.)

Easing the Transition

Having a plan in place takes a lot of pressure off both the child and the educators, since roles are defined, allowances and accommodations are outlined, and the method in which they are to be executed has been specifically stated. But, this is only the beginning. Over time, the 504 or IEP may need to be adjusted or updated as circumstances change. In the short term, there are other factors that must be addressed to ease the transition back to school.

After a long absence or hospitalization, your child may be dealing with more than just a backlog of schoolwork. Many of the drugs used to help control JA cause side effects that can affect their life at school. For example, steroids, a very common course of treatment, can cause significant weight gain and transform physical features. Earlier in the book, I shared a story about an instance when I didn't recognize my own child walking up to the car—and I had been living with him all that time!

When Grant was treated for his first serious flare, he was given massive doses of steroids, which he took in more moderate amounts for nearly six months. In the first three weeks, he went from an 85-pound preteen to a 130-pound child I hardly recognized. Although he gained a significant amount of weight, I was really shocked by how much it changed his facial features: He developed the classic "moon face" (facial roundness) and his eyes appeared smaller and more slanted. He had darker, more excessive facial and body hair, as well as a sensitive "hump" at the base of his neck. In medical terms, these changes are called *Cushing's syndrome*, but I would just say he looked like a different person.

Before Grant went back to school, his teacher made the other kids aware of these changes, to head off any shocked stares or innocent comments that might be hurtful. Having the other kids onboard really helped, and although there are always a few unexpected or cruel remarks, preparing the other children made a big difference in the emotional comfort level that Grant experienced at school. By preparing his classmates, my son had a much better chance of picking up his life closer to the way it was before. With the other kids treating him "like normal," he felt a little less self-conscious and could just be himself. In addition, allowing his classmates to ask all their questions *before* Grant returned helped to avoid many awkward conversations that inevitably would have taken place, as well as assuage the fears of his fellow students (and ultimately their parents), who worried about his condition being contagious.

Appearance is not the only drug-related issue your child may face, or that may need to be addressed with the school. Some medications can cause nausea or even require your child to make more frequent or urgent trips to the restroom. It's important to notify the school in advance, to save the child any undue embarrassment if a "situation" comes up rather suddenly that requires him or her to use the facilities prior to obtaining permission. Don't forget to also let your child know that, in these circumstances, they are allowed to excuse themselves! In my experience, most JA children try to be as normal as possible, thus masking their symptoms and needs so they don't get any special treatment from their teachers. Some may even worry about getting into trouble for taking care of their needs. If your child feels this way, it may be prudent to schedule a private meeting with the teacher or principal so the student knows exactly where he stands and what permissions are allowed in advance.

Another side effect of some rheumatology drugs is the onset of brain fog, which may make concentration more difficult. This is especially challenging in the school environment, as it directly affects your child's ability to focus, concentrate, and learn. You may even notice this brain fog at home, when your normally sharp child seems preoccupied, forgetful, spacey, or plagued by cloudy, illogical thought processes. You won't be able to fix this issue, but there are several things you can do to make it better.

Write Everything Down—If your child is old enough, encourage him or her to take notes and make lists to the best of their ability. Get written assignment sheets that outline what their tasks entail both during school and at home. If they're forgetful, they can refer back to the sheet.

Slow Down—Allow your child to take his or her time whenever possible. Being rushed through an assignment or hurried through speaking (kids can often forget a word or even what they were saying) will only make things worse, further reducing concentration. Be patient and encouraging. Although this won't cure cloudy thinking, it will prevent kids from getting flustered and allow them to get through the thought process on their own.

Avoid Multitasking Whenever Possible—If focus is an issue, help your child by concentrating on one thing at a time and reducing distractions.

Help Your Child Get Rest and Nutrition—As for any child, going to school on an empty stomach or being overtired can affect the ability to concentrate. Occasionally it may be necessary to allow your child to sleep in and get to school later, especially after a particularly challenging night or during a flare. It's better to have three quality hours of school than over six hours of worthless time due to brain fog!

Follow a Routine—A routine may help a child concentrate in an "autopilot" sort of way.

Look for a Brain Fog Pattern—Observe and track to see if a pattern can be established relative to the administration of medications. It may be possible to adjust the medication schedule so that the times your child has the highest mental clarity can be shifted to the hours spent at school. For example, if a once-a-day medication seems to cause memory issues for your child, it might be possible to switch its administration to nighttime rather than morning, making it easier to concentrate at school.

While challenging, learning to cope with a new set of circumstances *will* make your child stronger in the long run, helping him develop valuable life skills for handling adversity. In our case, Grant's ability to conquer his brain fog enough to function normally was a huge boost to his self-esteem. If he could accomplish things under those circumstances, nothing was going to stop him when he was 100 percent!

Have Realistic Expectations

It's important to remember that while your child may be the center of your life, he or she is one of many students in the classroom. Although the educators will try to do as much as possible for your child, keep your expectations realistic and don't demand an inordinate amount of time or resources to be allocated to your child. In some cases, a traditional public school setting may not work, and a smaller, private school, virtual school, or homeschool is the best option.

As I've said many times, there are no hard and fast rules or "one size fits all" scenarios when you're dealing with JA, which also applies to your child's education. What's right for him or her this year may not be the best option down the road. Case in point, during the last three years we have accessed services for hospital homebound instruction, traditional public schools, public education with a 504 plan, virtual school, *and* home school, as the situation warranted. By remaining open to all options and working with your current educational system, you can determine which services and types of education are best for your child and make adjustments as necessary.

SCHOOL STRATEGIES by RYAN MOLLET

For the past 11 years, I've had the good fortune of serving as a middle school principal, working with more than 1,500 students on a daily basis. It's been a very satisfying experience to help students reach success in both the academic and social domains. I've enjoyed watching students set and obtain academic goals, discover and explore scholarly interests, and establish friendships that may last a lifetime. I have learned, however, that the middle school experience is not easy for all students, especially those with a significant illness. In fact, the impact such an illness can have on a student's education can be considerable—influencing expected progress and limiting the traditional childhood experiences that regular attendance in school provides. I have found that stress, anxiety, and uncertainty are all typical responses parents may have when faced with this type of challenge. Based on my experience when working with this type of situation, I would suggest the following six strategies to help facilitate a successful school experience:

1. **Initiate a Meeting with the Building Principal**—As soon as you have a general diagnosis and the possible medical symptoms that may impede your child's ability and academic growth, contact the school's building principal. Ask for a face-to-face meeting with the intention of beginning effective and open communication with the school, as well as understanding and establishing the communication structure that will work best for all. Consideration should be given to weekly update meetings, establishing a lead contact, or group e-mails. While the best method of communication

may vary from school to school, the result should be the same: provide the right amount of information to the appropriate people.

2. Be Mindful of Your Audience—The tendency for parents to use medical terminology when communicating with the school team is understandable; however, this can be overwhelming for school personnel. When communicating with the school, parents should focus on their child's current condition. Talk about what he or she is capable of doing. Discuss his or her energy levels and ability to maintain the current schedule. Be sure to include social events and medical appointments. This will allow his or her teachers to establish appropriate academic expectations.

3. Explore School-Based Support Options—If your child is unable to attend school consistently, or his or her medical condition limits academic productivity, ask the principal (or appropriate school/district staff member) about creative support options that will help the student maintain academic progress. A few options to consider include:

- *Flexible Schedule* When examining a student's current state, the team could consider a flexible schedule that includes partial attendance or a modified day. For example, the student could attend morning classes one day and afternoon classes the next.
- *Homebound Tutoring* If the illness prohibits attendance altogether, the team should consider homebound tutoring, which allows the child to receive direct instruction in identified academic classes. Of course, each situation is different. Some

homebound experiences will maintain progress consistent with the school's curriculum objectives, while others will focus only on the essentials.

- *Section 504 Plan* In short, Section 504 of the Rehabilitation Act of 1973 is a law that protects the rights of a student with a qualifying disability. Oftentimes, a child with a significant illness that adversely impacts his or her education will qualify for educational services through a Section 504 plan. If a child is found eligible for support through this option, school-based accommodations will be established. These accommodations are student specific and determined by the educational team. For more information on Section 504 plans, visit the websites of your local school district, your state's Department of Education, or the U.S. Department of Education.

- *Individualized Education Program (IEP)* Similar to a Section 504 plan, an Individualized Education Program is a support plan designed to provide services to students with a qualifying disability. One of the differences between the two is that an IEP generally incorporates goals and objectives to measure a student's progress in a certain area. Again, the educational team will determine eligibility.

4. Maintain a Commitment to Academics— Generally speaking, school personnel will be inclined to put academics behind the student's medical needs. This certainly comes from a good place, as teachers simply want the child to get well. To the extent possible, maintain a commitment to academics. If a child is capable of completing some or all of the schoolwork, he/she should be required to do so. This will help maintain academic progress and ease reintegration into the school setting if an extended period of absence becomes necessary.

5. Maintain Social Experiences—In addition to academics, school has a very important social component. If a student does have to miss a significant amount of school, the potential for a delay in social progression becomes very real. To the extent possible, allow your child to attend birthday parties, playdates, school events, and other extracurricular activities. When considering a flexible schedule, perhaps your child could attend lunch at the school or an enrichment class that allows for social engagement.

6. Provide Coaching for Skills—Recognize the emotional impact that a significant illness and extended absences will have on your child and, if possible, provide coaching on the specific skills he or she may need to cope. When a student misses an extended period of school, he or she may experience a great deal of stress and/or anxiety. He or she may worry about work production, lack of understanding of the curriculum upon his or her return, or how social groups will respond to his or her inconsistent attendance. While it's impossible to plan for every situation that will surface, basic advocacy skills should be taught. These skills should focus on the student's ability to communicate with his or her teacher and respond to repeated questioning from his or her peer group about the illness or attendance pattern. Typically, schools have social workers on staff who could provide guidance to parents on how best to teach these skills, and if the student is well enough to attend school, they may be able to work with the student directly.

Of course, these are not the only strategies that will help promote a more successful school experience. They are, however, six options that have worked well for the students and parents with whom I've had the pleasure of working. While each situation is different and each school district is unique, the primary focus should always be on what's best for the student.

CHAPTER ELEVEN

The Whole Child

We've talked a lot about medical care and treating symptoms, which, of course, is a huge part of JA, but there is life outside the condition. Grant is still Grant, and Evan is still Evan—they aren't just "the Miller children with JA, poor things!" Evan is a soccer player and a fan of the game; he's a math whiz who loves video games and has a soft spot for animals. Grant loves all things sports, as well as travel and fishing. They are as different as night and day, and their disease does not define them. It's simply one aspect of their lives, not who they are.

It's an easy trap to fall into: JA becomes such a large part of your life that it gets entwined with your child's identity, or yours. But, JA should only be a part of your child's life, not the central focus. To me, "winning the game" against JA means raising the healthiest, happiest children I can, *in spite* of the disease. It means nurturing the whole child—mentally, emotionally, physically, and spiritually—despite the extra obstacles they face due to chronic illness. Winning is giving my children a real childhood that is not overshadowed by the additional challenges they face with JA.

What's Normal?

One of the best ways to protect their childhood is to make it as normal as possible. In order to do that, you must first define normal, which may differ for every family. What are you trying to accomplish? Are you trying to retain elements of your own childhood, or create a similar experience to the one enjoyed by your child's peers? In our case, we do use our children's peer group as the acid test for what our kids should be doing, but frame it within the morals and values of our own family practices.

Caring for their medical condition *and* letting them be children can be a difficult balancing act. We try to keep things as normal as possible, but make adjustments as the situation dictates. For example, our children are responsible for chores, even when they aren't "well." Everyone in our household has responsibilities. If our children are unable to do daily chores, then we find something they can do weekly, allow them more time, or permit them to suggest a job trade for something they *can* do. If they are unable to shovel the driveway, then they can clean the mirrors, put away dishes, and empty the wastepaper baskets instead. "Staying normal" means not allowing JA to become an excuse or a crutch. It means teaching them to cope and adjust.

Another big part of preserving normalcy is school. In our family, we believe that school for a child is the equivalent of a career for an adult: It's their "job" to attend. When they grow up, JA will still be a part of their lives, but they'll be expected to carry on and perform as a productive member of society, regardless. Beyond the obvious reasons for sending our children to school, we feel it's another way to maintain regularity in their daily lives and provide a training ground for what's to come in their future. This doesn't mean we send them to school regardless of their condition, but we do make every creative attempt possible to make it work, just as they would need to as adults. Overcoming the extra challenges they face, while still finding themselves able to perform academically at a level similar to their peers, provides a tremendous boost to their self-esteem. It has taught both my boys, but especially Grant, that they are far stronger (mentally and physically) than they may think. Ultimately, this gives them a drive to succeed and instills the "I *can* do it" mind-set far more than any coaching or lecturing could.

The Importance of Fun

Retaining as much of your usual day-to-day life as possible is important for your children, but forcing it too much can cause other problems. While normalcy may be your ultimate goal, getting there requires constant evaluation and adjustment to ensure you aren't setting unrealistic expectations or creating an environment that will cause undue psychological or emotional distress.

The truth is, as hard as we may try to create that "normal" environment for our kids, they *will* have many additional struggles and experiences that are out of the ordinary due to their illness. These things can take a heavy psychological toll, and it's important to try to balance their effects as much as possible. Maintaining an element of fun is crucial to fostering a normal childhood. If attending school full time is too taxing, then shoot for half days or early dismissal, with at least one fun extracurricular activity. If they're in clinic all day and miss school, still allow them the opportunity to play with a friend after school hours. Giving children something to look forward to and something to live for, within the context of what's important to *them*, is a critical element in preserving their psychological health. As important as it is to teach them to fulfill their responsibilities, it's equally important to give them a full, well-rounded life (within the limits of their abilities) that includes more than school, doctors, and chores. As children, they still need time to play, to have fun, to laugh and dream—making room for those activities also helps preserve a "normal" childhood.

Although the everyday activities are important, so are the once-in-a-blue-moon experiences. Before Grant was ill, we used to take two family vacations a year: one cold weather trip such as skiing and one warm adventure such as the beach. After he became ill, just leaving the house was a big ordeal, and travel was out of the picture (for a while anyway). The things we used to do and the way we used to do them seemed out of the question with our new circumstances, but travel was something that Grant *loved*, and the lack of it was definitely a source of angst. I was overwhelmed with all the new considerations I would need to make when traveling with him. We literally had a duffle bag full of *just* medications, many that required refrigeration. He was immunosuppressed and seemed to get sick any time he was around crowds (or in a crowded plane). He didn't have the stamina for many activities or extended car rides, but he was getting stir crazy! So what did we do? We learned to adjust.

We started taking short day or half-day trips planned around his good spells, taking advantage of what was in our own backyard—things we had never made time for in the past. When we were ready to venture a little further, we found out most hotels have mini-fridges *available at no charge* for medical purposes if you make arrangements in advance (medication problem solved!). We chose open-air activities (outside if possible) over crowded (germy) indoor excursions. We took the train instead of the car or plane, and traveled off-season, springing for our own private sleeper. We took meals in our cabin and enjoyed the view from our picture window. On a train, we had more room to move about, allowing Grant to walk the hall when he needed to stave off his stiffness. We had adventures that didn't tax him physically, while experiencing epic trips we wouldn't have discovered before. When we did need to take a plane, he wore a mask, and we scheduled much more flexibility and "rest" time into our schedules regardless of where we were or what we were doing. We have also learned to turn every trip (especially the medical ones) into a *travel* opportunity.

In addition to his wanderlust, Grant tends to be a bit of a foodie. When we have clinic visits that take us to downtown Chicago or Los Angeles, we make the most of the prospect. The evening before, he will use a service such as Yelp or Zagat or a website such as the Food Network to pick out a restaurant to try while we're there. Depending on how he's feeling, he may even choose to take in a famous sight or visit a museum, so our trips have more memories than just the inside of the hospital.

Planning these excursions also gives him something to anticipate, rather than approaching the upcoming visits with dread. Although he may not look forward to getting his labs drawn, or being examined *again*, at least it's balanced with something fun—something we would not have done without the clinic visit. Focusing on the good part of the visit helps him tolerate the not-so-great parts. What's more, these excursions don't have to be expensive to be enjoyable: the chosen "restaurants" have included food trucks and farmers' markets, and many of our adventures have been visits to friends who live close to the clinic (but far from us). Regardless, I make sure these activities are of Grant's choosing, not only to empower him, but also to make sure the "reward" is something meaningful to him.

TRAVEL TIPS

Traveling with kids can be challenging enough without the JA factor thrown in the mix! In addition to the usual considerations, families with chronically ill kids must address a number of important issues when taking any type of trip. Some things to keep in mind are:

Plan Frequent Rest Stops—Medications can cause kids to need more frequent restroom breaks, and JA can cause stiffness when staying in one position too long. Allow kids time to stretch and move around more frequently.

Modify Your Schedule to Consider Their Limitations—A full day at the theme park, going from dawn to dusk, can be a challenge for any child, but for a kid with JA, overexertion like this can result in one day of fun followed by three days in bed. Consider the use of a wheelchair if appropriate, or even half days at the park followed by an afternoon of lounging at the pool or enjoying another low key activity, such as movies in the hotel room.

Allow Plenty of Time for Rest and Recovery—Overtired children are a recipe for disaster anyway, but JA kids need their rest to recover from the additional activities, helping to avoid a potential flare.

Be Open to Changing Plans or Alternative Activities—JA can change a situation at the drop of a hat. Have an idea of the things you would like to do on your trip, but be willing to change your schedule if your child isn't up to it. Prior to your trip, research a number of alternate activities that could be fun if the original plans become impossible. On a recent trip to Orlando, we scrapped one day at Walt Disney World Resort for an opportunity to sit down for a few hours and take in an Orlando Magic game. For my little sports fans, this was a fair trade, and it allowed us to tone things down a bit, while staying within the same budget.

Pack All the Medical Supplies—In addition to packing all the medications, be sure to bring any medical device or equipment your child uses. Do they often use a heating pad or a cold pack? Do they occasionally use heel cups with increased walking? Do they use a TENS unit or other pain management device? It may seem inconvenient and cumbersome to bring everything along, but it beats ruining their trip if they need it and don't have it. Better safe than sorry.

Take Special Care with Medications—Pack all the meds your child will need for the duration of the trip with a couple extra days to spare. Make sure you have written down the pharmacy and prescription numbers, complete with dosages and refill dates, and tuck them in your wallet in case anything is lost, damaged, or stolen so it can be replaced. Consider investing in an insulated lunch bag or small cooler to transport medications. This way you can control the temperature and keep them with you, instead of leaving them in a hot car! Remember, most hotel rooms will provide a mini-fridge for medical purposes in your room, free of charge, with advance notification.

Know Which Medications Require Special Handling—If a medication must be refrigerated, an insulated bag with a cold or freezer pack will do the trick until you reach your destination. For longer trips (such as transoceanic flights), consider packing zippered plastic bags that the flight attendant can fill with ice to periodically replace your cold pack. Also, some medications should not go through the X-ray machine at the airport. Ask your pharmacist or contact the pharmaceutical company to see if any of the drugs your child takes should be hand checked. If you know you are traveling with a hand-check-only medication, be sure to tell your pharmacist when you have it refilled! We learned this lesson the *hard* way. Flying back from California, we had one of Grant's medications refilled at the local pharmacy. During the hand check (and wipe down), his medications tested positive for explosives! We were detained and tested, but came up clean. The analysis showed there were trace remnants of nitroglycerin (a common heart medication, which can also be found in explosives like dynamite!) on the box. It's likely that the pharmacist handled nitroglycerin and then touched our box. Several medications can cause this alert, so it's better to notify the pharmacy staff so they can take extra precautions to give you a "clean" container!

Keep a Few Snacks Handy—Nuts, dried fruit, or crackers are great choices for food "emergencies." While on vacation, mealtimes can vary while medication schedules do not. Keeping a few healthy snacks handy in your purse or backpack will ensure that you aren't caught empty-handed if meds "to be taken with food" are due. Make sure you pack enough to share with your "well" kids, too!

While traveling with JA kids can be more of a challenge, it's definitely worth the extra effort. We have our own war stories to share (which we typically look back on and laugh), but these travels have provided much-needed diversions from our day-to-day life and medical conditions. The vacations we have taken since JA are definitely different than those from our life before, but they are special in their own way, and we wouldn't trade those experiences either!

Empowering Your Child

Allowing Grant to choose how he will make the most out of clinic visits is not the only way we have empowered him. We've found that allowing him to make some decisions about his care and treatment plan and including him in many of the medical discussions have made him feel less helpless and more hopeful. Of course, your child's age and cognitive ability to make good decisions is an important part of determining how involved they can be, though we have found that even young children can benefit from feeling as though they have some control over their situation.

For very young kids, the decisions could be as simple as letting them decide which day of the week will always be "shot day," or which of the rotating injection sites they will choose for that day. It could be allowing them to take a couple of minutes at the beginning of their doctor's visit to tell the physician how *they* are feeling or what they are worried about. Since my children are older, some of the decisions they've helped to make include their participation in medical studies and the choice between two treatment plans offered by the medical team. Allowing them some opportunity for input empowers them to be an active participant in their treatment (it's much easier to get them to comply when they sign off on it!) and helps them to feel as though they are doing things *with* their team, rather than having things done *to* them.

Inclusion in the decision-making process is just one area in which you can empower your JA child. Another way is to foster their independence whenever possible. As tempting as it is to keep them as close as possible (I know, we all worry about the "what ifs" more with this disease), it's important to give them freedoms and developmentally appropriate opportunities to be self-sufficient. For older children, there are products on the market that can help them help themselves, such as the phone app My RA or a print version like *Body Check Journal*™ that help kids track their own symptoms.

If your child is old enough for a sleepover, you can test the waters by taking a hands-off approach at your own home first. Administer meds; provide a safe, secure environment; and then remain hands off unless they come to you (or you realize something non-medical needs checking) until the next morning. If your child makes it through the evening without incident, it may be time to let them try a sleepover away from home.

Although Grant had been participating in sleepovers for years, after he was diagnosed he started taking so many medications and had so many health issues that could change instantly that I was hesitant to have him leave the house on his own for any amount of time! Knowing he needed to regain some independence, I found a short, stay-away camp (just four days and three nights) that also had a nurse on staff who was willing to take on his "case." Since it was a camp focused on one of Grant's interests (not a JA camp), they requested we provide a release form that would allow them to take him to the hospital if necessary, along with the name of a local doctor they could contact. As an extra precaution, they also requested that I stay within a distance that would allow me to reach the camp within two hours. I had further prepared him with a boy's Med-icAlert® necklace (which could be hidden under his shirt) that was linked to a current electronic record of all his medications and an app on his phone to document his symptoms. Truthfully, both of us were a little nervous, but the week went off without a hitch, and he had a fantastic time!

After a successful camp experience, I also permitted Grant to resume sleepovers, even allowing him to travel to visit friends who had moved across the country. I made sure that I trusted the parents who accepted the responsibility and provided them with a written list of his doctors, diagnoses, medications, and medication schedule. These outings were nearly as good for his *total* recovery as any new drug or treatment. As he continues to get better, we are constantly figuring out new ways for him to experience life independently and more opportunities for him to safely spread his wings.

Caring for Their Spirit

Regardless of your beliefs, spirituality, or religion, you will find that dealing with a chronic, potentially fatal illness causes you to question and dig deep. Children, especially as they get older, are no different. As they recognize that bad things have been happening to them, for no fault of their own, they will undoubtedly begin to ask difficult questions.

In some instances, the greatest gift you can give them is a qualified, caring third party to listen and advise them. They are your kids, after all, and let's face it, much of what parents say goes in one ear and out the other. Meanwhile, hearing the same advice from someone else can have an impact. This "someone else" may be another kid who has lived through these issues and come out okay on the other side. It may be a licensed therapist or counselor, or it might be a spiritual advisor through your place of worship. Older kids might ask why God would do something like this to them, and while it may be easier to gloss over their concerns, it's important to address their questions. In Grant's case, handling this delicate question with thoughtfulness and compassion has strengthened his faith in some areas, although he still struggles in others. Nurturing the spiritual aspect of your child's life within the context of your family's beliefs can be a tremendous comfort to all but the very youngest of children, and should not be overlooked in your care of the *whole* child.

Dealing with Burnout

Despite our best efforts to prevent it, dealing with a chronic illness can often result in burnout, even in very young children. We do whatever we can to give them the life they used to have within the context of their new normal, but at some point every child who deals with a chronic illness will want to throw their hands up and say, "No more! I quit!"

Burnout can be a very serious issue. It may result in behavioral issues or noncompliance with treatments and, at its worse, may cause children to contemplate or attempt suicide. Regardless of where your child may fall within that spectrum, burnout is a very important concern that should be addressed as soon as it's recognized. Some of the warning signs that your child may be feeling burnout include:

- depression
- defeatist attitude
- loss of their "zest" for life
- lack of interest in friends or former pursuits
- increasing expression of "disappointment"
- reduced functioning within their physical capabilities
- resistance to comply with treatments/clinic visits
- behavioral issues (quick to anger or cry, increasing resentment, etc.)

If you feel as though your child is beginning to experience these symptoms, it's crucial to seek out help and work with your child to alleviate some of these feelings. Take time to *really* listen to what your child has to say. Take notes if you need to, and then address each of his or her concerns. Being "heard" can help children cope. Even if they don't get the resolution they're looking for, they know they have a voice and are being taken seriously. When Grant had gained so much weight from his medications, he was very depressed and did not want *any* pictures taken. Although we complied with his request for the most part, there were still a few photos that ended up sneaking in, usually including a part of him in the background when we were photographing his brother. When Grant was at his wits end, I dug up those pictures so he could see how far he really *had* come. Then we made an appointment with the pediatrician and let him know that this concern was Grant's first priority. The doctor listened. Shortly after, Grant was seen by an endocrinologist, who determined that he *did* have a medical issue that was previously unrecognized, causing him to retain far too much weight. Once we addressed that problem, in a short time Grant began to look and feel more like his "old" self. And because he had been heard, he was back to working with me *and* the doctors.

Another way to prevent or alleviate burnout is to cut back on any of the activities that are causing undue stress. Is your child being pushed too hard and too fast to attend long hours at school? Could doctors' appointments or labs be consolidated for fewer appointments? Can some specialists' exams or requests be covered by other doctors, scheduled less frequently, or even dropped unless an issue arises? Are all the tests really necessary, or can some be avoided?

Over time, we have found that we don't *need* to know everything if the answers won't change the treatment plan. For instance, Grant's one-year follow-up for a recommended repeat esophagogastroduodenoscopy (EGD), a test that involves inserting a camera into the esophagus, was tabled because his symptoms were subsiding (although not gone), and the medications he was taking would not change, regardless of the results. Instead of putting him through another procedure at the standard time for follow-up, Grant's gastroenterologist agreed we could avoid the test unless there were physical signs the situation had changed for the worse. Although the worrywart in me would have loved the confirmation, the mom in me knew that avoiding as many of these borderline necessary tests was the *best* thing I could do for Grant at the time. I also had faith in the ability of our team to closely monitor his health for changes without these invasive tests. Telling him he could delay, or possibly avoid, an "icky" procedure was almost as good as winning the lottery!

Reducing the stress load (where possible) is only part of the equation. It's also important to help your child regain the activities that bring joy into their lives—things they may be missing after diagnosis. Many times, the doctors will recommend cutting back or eliminating certain activities. However, sometimes compromises can be made to modify these activities so your child can participate in the things he or she truly enjoys. Parents can make compromises, too. For example, we used to strictly limit "screen time," but after Grant became ill, we found that Facebook, Xbox Live, Skype, and Facetime were great ways for him to stay connected with his friends, even if he wasn't well enough to meet with them face-to-face.

In the battle against burnout, don't underestimate the power of positive thinking. It's important to be our children's most supportive cheerleaders! Remind them how brave they have been, how much you admire them, and how proud you are. Find ways to boost their morale and ego. The photos I have from the worst times compared to those taken more recently, during better times, help Grant remember just how far he has come. I have told him many times that he is braver than I was at his age. I admire him for the difference he is making in other people's lives, using his disease as a platform to do good.

Finally, I would recommend spending more quality time as a family whenever possible, reminding each other of the silver lining in every difficult situation. We have made very dear friends who may have never crossed our paths if not for meeting them through our medical journeys. Grant may have lost a few friends along the way, but his friendships have been strengthened with those worth having. We have taken trips and had experiences that we never would have considered if not for the allowances we were forced to make. Going through these tremendously hard times with Grant has developed a special bond and trust between us, while instilling empathy in Evan that could never be replicated without those experiences. We have developed more flexibility and learned to embrace change, as well as found ways to be grateful for so much more in our lives—proving that caring for the "whole child" can strengthen the whole family.

JA will attempt to take over as soon as it makes that first unwanted entrance into your family's lives. It is not a force to be ignored, and it will make its mark on every aspect of your child's life, but it doesn't have to win. You can turn the negative experiences into positive life lessons. You can use JA to make your kids stronger. You can recognize what it can do and plan your counterattack against it; allowing your children to be kids first and JA patients second!

LIFE LESSONS by GRANT

Life with arthritis is hard. If I had to describe it with one word, it would be *frustrating*.

For a while, I knew things just weren't right, but I didn't really know what was wrong. I could tell that I wasn't myself and things that used to be easy were getting harder. I had pain and didn't feel as well as I once felt, even when I was supposed to be healthy. It was confusing and frustrating. I didn't know what was happening or why, but it occurred so gradually at first that I tried to just live with it.

As I began to feel worse and my mom noticed more of my symptoms, I thought the situation would improve. I was sure that once we had a diagnosis things would get better, since we would know what to do and how to fix it. But, the truth is that's when I became the most frustrated.

When I found out that I had juvenile arthritis, I had a lot of mixed emotions. I was relieved to find out that I wasn't crazy—there were *real* reasons for the way I was feeling, and we finally knew the cause. But, I was also sad to know I had an incurable disease. I was scared and angry. I wondered how I would play sports, go to school, and do all the other little things in everyday life. I knew some people who had arthritis (such as my dad and grandparents with osteoarthritis), so I also knew how much it could hurt. I was afraid that having arthritis would prevent me from realizing my dreams of playing in the NFL like my dad. Then, when I was told that the type of arthritis I had was totally different from osteoarthritis, I was even more confused. I didn't know what to think, and the not knowing made me worry even more.

Every part of your life has good and bad parts, but it seemed like JA was causing frustration in every single area of mine. I was frustrated by:

- **Doctors**—Even though I know they were trying, I was frustrated by how long it took to figure out my case and how to treat it properly. The doctors knew what was wrong, but couldn't seem to keep me from suffering for a long time. They didn't have answers to my questions, and sometimes it seemed as though some of them just weren't trying their hardest, while I had to live with it. I got tired of telling the same story over and over to lots of different doctors—all of whom had to see me or observe a certain symptom several times before they believed me anyway.
- **Medicine**—While I wanted the doctors to find something I could

take that would help me get my old life back, I still hated taking so much medicine. I was discouraged by the way the medication made me feel—some made me feel worse than the disease! Due to side effects and allergic reactions, I never felt "well," and sometimes felt worse. Some medications made things harder (like I couldn't be in the sun or eat because they made me violently nauseated). Many times I traded one symptom for another. I was frustrated that the medications helped me control the disease, but I wasn't feeling better. In fact, sometimes the medications made me feel like I was suffering with *another* disease! I never had any time, day or night, for over a year when I just felt perfectly well.

- **People**—I was frustrated with adults who didn't understand what I was going through, and talked about me like I couldn't hear them (saying I was faking or taking advantage of the situation). Some people were *sure* I would grow out of it or that I could do better. I was also upset that some of the other kids, not just the mean kids, but also my friends, forgot about me because I wasn't around as much in school or sports—or didn't include me because I had to cancel so many times. It made me feel alone; like no one understood.

- **School**—I simply did not feel well enough to go to school a lot of the time. Because of that, I was losing ground academically and worried that I might have to repeat a grade or look like I wasn't smart anymore. Then I worried that I wouldn't be ready for high school and not performing well there could affect my whole life through college. It was frustrating to think that even trying my hardest may not be enough to be successful. I felt like I was losing control even though none of this was my choice or my fault.

- **Family**—I was frustrated that some family members didn't understand. Sometimes my parents pushed me too hard or my brother assumed I was exaggerating for attention. Sometimes relatives who didn't see me as often would get irritated because one day I could do something and then the next day or later that day I couldn't. My cousins would get annoyed with *me* when I was too tired to play more than 15 minutes of basketball with them, because I used to play for two hours. It felt as though no one really understood what I was going through.

- **Weight**—While I was on steroids, I gained a lot of weight. It made me slow and not able to perform as well in sports. It made my back, knees, and ankles hurt on top of the arthritis. It made people treat me differently. Three weeks after I got out of the hospital and was trying to start playing baseball again, I was so bloated from the steroids that it was hard to find a uniform that fit me. Even after I found one, I knew I looked terrible. I tried to be brave and get out there even though I knew people would probably say things. Sure enough, when I got up to bat, one of the parents said, "Well, he looks like he's had one too many ho-hos!" and the crowd laughed. I was so upset and hurt that I could barely stay at the plate. I had a pinch runner because I wasn't well enough to run yet, but I knew I could be in the field and bat, so I had gotten into a "friendly" noncompetitive league as a way to get some of my "fun" activities back. But after that comment, I didn't want to leave the house for almost a week. I was frustrated because I hardly recognized myself in the mirror, and people didn't see *me* anymore. They saw someone to make fun of or feel sorry for.

- **Height**—I used to be one of the tallest kids in my class, but then I got sick and my growth just stopped. Some docs thought it was due to the steroids, others thought it was caused by the inflammation from my disease, and still others thought it was a combination of both. Either way, I pretty much stopped growing at about 4 feet 11 inches. Both my parents are tall, and my younger brother and all my friends were getting bigger than me. That was really hard in middle school! It was also frustrating because I want to play sports, just like my dad, and the lack of growth was one more thing that might keep me from getting there, through no fault of my own.

- **Sports**—Before I got sick, I was one of the star players, but with JA I had to work ten times harder just to get a spot off the bench. I felt like I let my team down, and that I would never be good enough to move to the next level, or eventually the NFL. The one thing I loved so much and dreamed about the most was becoming less and less likely. Sports are a big part of who I am, and I felt they were getting taken away from me.

Basically, nothing was fun anymore and every single part of my life was getting ruined by JA. *Everything*! It was so much more than being sick and having pain. There was nothing in my life that it didn't try to ruin, *nothing* that it didn't affect—sports, school, family, friends, health, appearance—nothing was the same. But you know what? I didn't let JA win. Not then, and not now.

Although this disease continues to frustrate me, I refuse to let it run my life. I started the worst chapter of my life with JA when I was 11, and now that I am almost 15, I know it has taught me a lot and can't keep me down.

I have learned to talk to the doctors and tell them what's frustrating, as well as letting them know when their plan is not acceptable to me. Often, they can offer a compromise, or at least better explain to me why they can't, and that helps me to be less frustrated with them.

I have started to educate the people who say things they shouldn't or know nothing about this disease. I approach my friends to do things when I can, rather than wait for them to include me. I have developed a thicker skin so I'm not as sensitive to stupid comments. After all, those comments are a reflection of the people who say them, not me. I can be proud of myself because I know what I'm accomplishing and what I've overcome: I don't need someone else to verify that to make it real.

I'm not afraid to let my family know how it is; if they don't get it, I'll explain it to them, or I'll let the people who do understand help educate others for me. I don't let other people pressure me into doing stuff that will make *them* happy (like playing too much basketball) when I know it will be bad for me. They love me, so eventually they start to understand—I just have to keep reminding them.

My height and weight don't worry me as much now, since the doctors found out what was causing these problems and things are starting to get better. Even though it meant I had to add more doctors and new medications, I feel like I'm on the right track. Being short and heavy for a while taught me a few things. It showed me that some people can be mean, but I also learned not to take things so hard and that what these people say really doesn't matter. It also revealed who my real friends were, and who had good character, even for adults. Finally, I learned firsthand how hard it can be when you're different. After I had to deal with this, I became a lot more vocal against bullying or saying mean things. Before, I might not speak up if someone said something unkind, but now I don't allow anyone to say anything mean about another kid around me, whether that kid can hear it or not. It taught me to make a difference wherever I can and to have more empathy. You never know a person's whole story and you can't be the judge.

Where sports are concerned, I learned a lot as well. I have more appreciation for where I am since I had to work really hard to get back to where I was. I never had to go the extra mile to be one of the "great" kids before, but now I do. And, I have seen how much better I can be by going the extra mile, even if I'm already one of the best. Even the best players can improve! I always wanted to work hard, but now I am even more driven to work my hardest. Nothing can stop me. I even went with my team and played GOOD football at the AYF national championship tournament in Orlando, Florida, while I was taking a chemo drug! I may have thrown up on the sideline, but I still earned my spot, and my talent was underestimated by my opponents. We didn't go all the way, but getting as far as we did, doing so well, and earning my place despite all the additional obstacles in my way was one of the best feelings ever!

I also came to realize that not being able to play sports doesn't mean I can't still be active in sports. When I was too sick to play, I learned how to announce a game and even went to sports broadcasting camp. I was paid to be a junior umpire for baseball and had a couple announcement gigs in Little League play-offs. I even helped assistant coach the seven-year-old team for our area's football organization. After taking a mandatory season off sports, I came back better than ever and stronger. At first it was hard, because I wanted to be the one out there, but when I was able to come back I found I was even better. I wanted it more, so I achieved more. When I returned to baseball, I hit my first home run and it was a grand slam!

Of course, all these things happened over three years, which didn't seem fast enough at the time, so I was still a little frustrated. But, when I look back, I appreciate all these experiences and everything they taught me—the patience I gained, the way I learned to speak up for myself, and the way I learned how to make lemonade out of lemons. When these things were happening, it made me feel really unhappy and frustrated, but now I understand the lessons that will help me so much in life. There are many adults who haven't learned these lessons yet!

To all the other kids out there with JA or another chronic illness, I would say this: use it to your advantage. There are things you can learn from it and experiences you wouldn't have if it wasn't part of your life. Look at me: I learned to announce, umpire, and coach. If it weren't for JA, I wouldn't have taken the time to do those things. I would have just been playing and not appreciating how lucky I was. I learned to stand up for myself and take the chances that I could. I learned to do things for myself, instead of waiting for my mom, my coach, or my teacher to get it for me. I learned to work harder than I needed to and that the results made *me* the happiest. Best of all, I learned to be happy without letting the frustrations get the best of me. And, you can, too

CHAPTER TWELVE

Too Many Hats

Chances are you wear many hats, including medical caregiver, social worker, educator, and therapist—not to mention mom (or dad), which encompasses nurturer, chauffeur, cook, maid, and many other "jobs." Sometimes the roles we play seem endless! It's easy to get lost in what everyone else expects you to be or wants you to be ... but what about YOU?

You've probably heard it a million times, but it's true: When you're taking care of someone else (or several others), it's still important to take care of *yourself*. I'm not suggesting you dump your sick kid for a solo vacation to Tahiti, as tempting as that may sound at times. What I mean is you need to pay enough attention to your emotional and physical health so you can continue to be there and stay strong for your family—because they *all* need you, not just the sick ones! The way you handle the stress and demands that accompany JA will affect the way others around you handle them as well, especially your child. Your well-being will affect the mood and "feeling" of your home environment, increasing or reducing tensions. Your approach will affect the way the medical community views you and deals with you. In other words, your attitude can be a great asset or a huge liability throughout this journey. The challenge becomes figuring out what works best to help *you* get and stay in a "good place."

Let's Get Real

I want to be realistic here. No one can go day after day, week after week, year after year without backsliding a little. It's normal to feel like throwing your hands up in the air and quitting! It's common to feel the need to submit to a good cry, hold your own pity party once in a while, or occasionally have a short fuse. However, it's not okay to get stuck there! It's healthy to give in to those feelings from time to time, in a way that can be controlled and worked through, and then move on. Although you may recognize this is happening to your child and have addressed many of these very same issues with them, it's a big part of your life as well. You'll find yourself going through many of the same emotions. It's important to acknowledge these feelings and deal with them before they get out of hand, but allow them to run their course. No one can play Pollyanna forever, and that isn't healthy either. Allow yourself to grieve— for your child, for yourself, and for the changes that are inevitable.

Your life will never be the same. Once you accept that, you can figure out how to make the most of it. Learning to alleviate stress, cope with the changes, and work through the negative feelings are necessary before you can enjoy life and get back on track. That may sound impossible, but trust me, it will happen—you can and will enjoy your life again! Remember, you're on that trip to Holland even though you planned for Italy. Once you adjust your expectations, you can harness the power of positive thinking again. Even though your child has JA, you can still be happy, and so can they. The journey is just a bit more challenging, with bigger peaks and valleys along the way.

Making It Happen

In the most simplistic of explanations, you have to identify what makes you happy, and conversely what makes you unhappy. Then add in more of the "happy" things whenever you can, even if they're small! For example, do fresh flowers boost your mood? Buy some, or clip a few from your yard, and enjoy the mood-boosting effects every time they catch your eye. How about wearing perfume, even when you aren't leaving the house all day, or throwing a batch of slice-and-bake cookies in the oven before the kids get home from school? It's great to luxuriate in those wonderful smells, or be the hero with a plate of warm cookies. These things don't have to be huge or expensive, but surrounding yourself with mood lifters and making small efforts to brighten the day can add up to big results.

By the same token, removing as many "unhappy" triggers as possible can also help improve your and your child's outlook. Grant could not stand looking at his medications every time he passed the kitchen counter. Those vials were foreshadowing the many shots and pills to come, as well as reminding him of how sick he was. Both our attitudes improved when I cleared out a small corner cabinet to "hide" the medications until they were needed. Happier kid equals a happier mom, simple. For me, leaving the bills out on the desk caused anxiety every time I looked at the stack. So, one day I decided to put them in a drawer and address them at a determined time. I didn't stop paying the bills; I simply removed the constant reminder.

I challenge you to sit down and write a list of ten small things that make you happy and ten small things that do not (things that are in your power to change in the next 48 hours). Think really small and doable. Then attack that list. See the difference? Small changes can create an environment that positively affects your attitude and promotes happiness. The things that work (or don't work) will be unique to you, but I can offer some suggestions that may help, or at least give you a little insight into what worked for me.

- **Rely on Your Support Systems**—Having a child (or two) diagnosed with a serious chronic disease precipitates a major life change. Now is the time to utilize the support systems you have built. Talk to the friend or family member who actually *listens*. Vent to other parents who are going through (or have been through) the same things via online forums for tried-and-true advice. Make it easy on yourself and don't reinvent the wheel!
- **Give Yourself a Break**— If it's a day when all the kids can

actually go to school, don't fill it up with chores. Sometimes the vacuuming or laundry needs to wait so you can take a hot bath or read a book for 30 minutes. Most families can survive putting off the laundry for a couple of hours or a day! Spend those few found minutes to catch up on the TV series you've been recording or the current activity on your Facebook newsfeed ... whatever your "escape" may be. It's not self-indulgent; it's supporting your own mental health. I'm not advocating losing yourself for hours, but rather taking a little time to refresh and recharge your batteries—even if it's only 5–10 minutes at a time sprinkled through the day. It's a way to mentally "step away" for a bit and lose the ever-present thoughts about illness. Find a way to laugh, or take a nap so you're ready for the next long night. When you take a break you may find your perspective has changed for the better again.

- **Lose the Guilt and Quit Worrying**—Sure, it's easier said than done, but guilt and worry can drain you of time and energy. What's done is done, and guilt only holds you in the past. We have all done things wrong, even when we're trying our hardest. We can't control everything, but we often make ourselves crazy trying. Letting yourself get lost in these emotions will only cripple your ability to handle what's coming next. Recognize the mistakes you've made and learn from them; let them empower you for the next set of challenges because now you know better. Work through the concerns you have for your child and his or her illness, not by getting stuck worrying over what can happen, but by being realistic about the possibilities and then preparing for them. Choose to be happier, and don't give into the things that steal your happiness!

- **Consider Counseling**—If making changes on your own isn't enough, or you find yourself struggling with your emotions, you may find counseling helpful. Whether it's long term or a few sessions to help you develop coping techniques, a qualified professional can help you work out your feelings while providing some objectivity. You can choose to have individual sessions or include other family members.

The important thing is to recognize that you have needs, too, and you must find a way to address those needs so you can stay strong for others. You are in the driver's seat!

SHADES of GUILT by SARAH

Among the many emotions parents experience when faced with a chronically ill child, guilt ranks high on the list. Guilt is defined as an emotional experience that occurs when a person realizes or believes—whether justified or not—that he or she is responsible for some violation or wrong: a conflict that occurs when we feel we've done something we shouldn't, or conversely, haven't done enough. Since my daughter, Emma, was diagnosed with JA, I have struggled with guilt in many forms.

"Who Done It" Guilt

When I first found out my sweet child was afflicted by some disease I had never heard of, the burning question was "Why?" I found myself asking, *"Why my baby?" "Why now?" "Why? Why? Why?"* Yet no one had an answer. There is no obvious reason for the pain and suffering my child has had to endure.

Of course, that's not acceptable to a parent's ears—there must be *some* reason.

In came the guilt, as I began to wonder if this disease was my fault.

After all, I provided half of her genetic makeup, carried her in my womb for nine months, breast-fed her, and chose her food from the store. Logical or not, I went through a great deal of guilt wondering if JA was caused by something I had done, or not done. Thankfully, I moved beyond this notion, but it's very common for parents to feel this way after a scary diagnosis.

"To Medicate or Not" Guilt

After a diagnosis of juvenile arthritis, the next step is to come up with a treatment plan. Depending on the type of JA, treatment may involve some frightening medication options, including chemotherapy drugs, immune suppressants, and steroids. These meds can cause a variety of serious side effects and make our kids more susceptible to infection. *What if my baby develops cancer because I chose to give her these drugs? What if she becomes sterile and can't have children of her own? What if she gets a rare infectious disease and ends up in the hospital?*

With each new medication, the same fears resurface. And, along with these questions comes the guilt. However, the alternative is *not* to medicate. Choosing not to treat JA with these medications could result in permanent joint damage, which means my child may be unable to walk, tie her shoes, or even hold a pencil. *How long before she will need surgery to replace a knee or hip? How long will she be able to endure the chronic pain?*

"Administering Meds" Guilt

So, every day I choose to administer drugs that will ease my child's pain and maintain mobility, while threatening her liver, or worse. Sometimes I'm lucky, and she takes her meds like a champ. Other times, she thinks it's "gross" and fights me every step of the way.

Every week, my daughter also receives an injection to decrease her inflammation and enable her to walk, while putting her at higher risk for organ damage and infection. Again, sometimes she screams and cries, forcing my husband to hold her down while she receives the injection. On other days, she sits still and is proud of herself for being brave. But, since she is only two years old, she shouldn't have to be this brave—which, of course, leads to more guilt.

"My Baby Is Sick" Guilt

Emma woke up with a cough one Sunday morning, so I kept her home from church and took her temperature multiple times. When it was time for her to take her JA meds, I had a decision to make: should I give her these drugs or wait? Since Emma didn't have a fever, she got her injection, as usual. Later that night, her cold became worse and she developed a fever. *Is this just the natural progression of the virus, or is it worse because I gave her those immune suppressing drugs? Should I have held off giving her these injections until the cold passed?* Every time my kid catches a cold, flu, or bizarre viral rash, I think to myself, *"Maybe this infection/cough/fever wouldn't be so severe if I had just skipped her dose of medication this week."* More guilt.

We've been very lucky. Emma has had some nasty bugs since starting JA medication, but she's managed to stay out of the hospital and, overall, remains in good health. Which leads me to my last category ...

"My Baby Is Doing So Well!" Guilt (aka "Remission" Guilt)

At the beginning of this journey, I felt alone. My family was completely isolated with this horrible disease and an unknown future before us. So we reached out and made friends with other JA families. They have been a huge source of strength, love, and support.

In getting to know other parents of JA kids, I have come to realize that we are blessed. Emma's JA has affected fewer than ten joints. Her eyes and internal organs have been spared so far. She was diagnosed quickly and began treatment right away. She responded beautifully to her medication and hasn't had a new flare since the initial onset of this disease. We haven't seen any active arthritis in an entire year! She is in medicated remission! This is wonderful!

Yet, I feel guilty that my daughter is doing so well when some of my friends' children suffer continually, are in and out of hospitals, and get a seemingly endless amount of bad news from doctors. *Why can't they have the same success we have been able to enjoy?*

I have heard guilt referred to as a waste of energy—it doesn't help the situation or change the outcome. However, for many JA families, it's a very real part of living with this disease. All we can do is learn to deal with these emotions effectively so they don't wear us down. Feelings of guilt may come and go, but JA never goes away.

The Health Factor

When you're caring for a sick child, it's easy to neglect your own health. Lack of sleep, poor eating habits, and stress can take a toll over time. Additionally, after spending so many hours at doctors' offices and clinics with your child, the last thing you want to do is make an appointment for yourself. Many caregivers forgo regular checkups, but it's important to look after your own physical health. If you let yourself get too run down, not only will you be grumpy and less able to handle things, but you also run the risk of getting sick and being no good to anyone! Considering that most JA kids on medications are immunosuppressed, your being sick can be even *more* problematic for everyone.

Diet and Exercise

Make sure you're eating quality foods as regularly as possible, staying hydrated, and balancing rest and exercise as well as possible under your unique circumstances. Where there's a will, there's a way. Having a child in the hospital can be exceptionally challenging, but with a little creative thinking you can still help yourself in these areas. When staying at the hospital with my son, I was physically and mentally exhausted, eating out of the vending machines, and sitting in a chair most of the time. Those unhealthy circumstances only compounded things, during a time that was hard to feel good anyway!

Following my roomie mom's lead, I started taking the stairs to the vending area, sprinting up all five flights when I could. And, you know what? I ended up with more energy. I also felt some of that pent-up stress and anger melt away. When my husband came in the evenings, I asked him to pack me a healthy meal from home, instead of relying on hospital food. These small changes helped me take better care of myself in a less-than-ideal environment. Later, I knew if I could do it at the hospital, I could do it at home.

I began parking in the farthest spot from the pharmacy or grocery store entrance and did a few push-ups here and there at home. It wasn't the gym, but these tiny efforts helped keep me active and healthy until my life was more on track again. Don't be overwhelmed by the thought of having to devote a large amount of time to exercise, or you may end up doing nothing at all. Studies show that short bouts of exercise throughout the day are beneficial, so even a 10 to 15 minute walk around the block can give you a healthy boost. The key is figuring out what you *can* do for yourself, and then doing it.

Stress

Diet and exercise are not the only components to staying healthy. Stress can also impact your health. Of course, a certain amount of stress is unavoidable, but if left unchecked, high stress levels have been proven to be physically damaging to your body. Because of these effects, there are hundreds of books available to help you address the issue. Personally, I have learned to lessen the effects of stress by streamlining my life and learning to let go. It's also helpful to distinguish between true "needs" versus "wants," and then getting rid of the clutter in your life. I don't mean disposing of actual stuff (although some folks do find that cathartic); I'm referring to losing the unnecessary things that take up your time and energy. In fact, I can't emphasize this enough.

There were so many activities and obligations that used to fill our time before the "big change" after Grant's first hospitalization. In the beginning, I really tried to keep up with everything in our old life—and subsequently made myself crazy. In time, I learned that ironing Evan's shirt before school and having a hot two-course breakfast waiting for him when he bounded down the stairs were not requirements. He didn't *need* a homemade lunch packed every single day (and, in fact, he preferred school lunches on Mondays and Fridays). He needed my attention more than these other things, and cutting out the fluff allowed me to give him more of my time. Serving a bowl of oatmeal instead of a fancier, labor-intensive meal gave me a few extra minutes to sit at the table and have my coffee *with* him while he ate breakfast, and linger longer on the days I didn't pack lunch.

I discovered the world wouldn't end if I slept in an extra ten minutes (I love my snooze button!) and ran the kids to school without putting on my makeup. I didn't have to make time for tea with each of my friends every time I was invited or be a regular at Bible study. All these things in my old routine (which used to be enjoyable, except for the ironing!) just added pressure under our new circumstances. Streamlining was surprisingly liberating. Now that my little people are doing somewhat better,

PUT THE GLASS DOWN

While teaching a class on stress management, a psychologist raised a glass of water to the audience. Naturally, everyone expected they'd be asked the "half empty or half full" question. Instead, with a smile on her face, she inquired, "How heavy is this glass of water?"

The students called out answers ranging from 8 to 20 ounces.

But the psychologist dismissed them all by replying, "The absolute weight doesn't matter. It depends on how long I hold the glass. If I hold it for a minute, it's not a problem. If I hold it for an hour, I'll have an ache in my arm. If I hold it for a day, my arm will feel numb and paralyzed. In each case, the weight of the glass doesn't change, but the longer I hold it, the heavier it becomes."

She continued, "The stresses and worries in life are like that glass of water. Think about them for a while and nothing happens. Think about them a bit longer and they begin to hurt. And if you think about them all day long, you will feel paralyzed—incapable of doing anything."

It's important to remember to let go of your stresses. As early in the evening as you can, put all your burdens down. Don't carry them through the evening and into the night. Remember to put the glass down!

I have added a few of those activities back into my life, but I realized that many things just made me busier than I had to be.

I learned to say *No*. I traded rigid commitments for similar activities that allowed for more flexibility. I didn't have to bake for *every* bake sale or chaperone every field trip, and I found it was perfectly acceptable to order pizza instead of cooking every now and again. So what if I always had two or three loads of laundry waiting instead of an empty laundry room? As long as everyone always had clean clothes, then I could let some of that go. Did my husband or friends really judge me for the state of my laundry room? Of course not. I was doing that to myself. Now I just shut the door—problem solved.

Of course, I recognize that, for some people, leaving things undone can cause more stress, but for me, giving myself a little latitude was just what the doctor ordered, and you know what? Everyone survived, and I learned to *breathe*. I accepted that I couldn't control everything and began to focus on the things that I could. I dealt with issues that really needed attention, while allowing some of the less important things to slide. I was much happier, and so was my family!

Knowledge Is Power

During the early days, my stress levels were often directly linked to the perceived lack of control concerning Grant's condition. Educating myself helped me to feel more in control. The more I knew, even if it was scary, the less I was frightened of the unknown. By learning about most of the possible case scenarios, medications, and plausible outcomes, I was able to think through realistic plans of action and not be surprised by bad news. When I had an idea of what would or could happen, nothing hit me like a ton of bricks anymore. If we avoided something bad, I was even more thankful and happy, since I had already been informed of that potential. It helped me celebrate each of the small medical victories and to keep hope alive. If we did get the "bad" news, I was no longer shocked and numb, because I already had questions formed and had worked out that possibility in my head.

HOW TO SEARCH THE INTERNET

The Internet is filled with information—**not all of it accurate**. Although it can be a tremendous help and excellent resource, it can also provide dangerous misinformation if not used with caution. Most parents who find themselves caring for a chronically ill child with a diagnosis such as JA do not have a background in medicine or research, making it difficult to determine which sources should be trusted, or even how to look. Some tips to keep in mind as you search the Internet include:

- **Consider the Source**—Begin your search utilizing reputable sources such as the NIH, foundation websites (such as the Arthritis Foundation), and PubMed or Medline. If you want to do a Google search, consider using Google Scholar, which returns academic results.

- **Focus Your Search**—Break a large subject, such as JA, into smaller, more specific topics to make your search manageable. If your search is too broad, you will be overwhelmed. Pick a few key terms and expand from there. Consider using medical subject headings (MeSH) terminology for a more targeted approach. For a tutorial, access www.nlm.nih.gov/bsd/disted/meshtutorial/.

- **Confirm the Sources**—If you happen across a nonacademic article, check the sources and look at the primary research. Double check these findings through PubMed or online libraries.

- **Take It Back to the Doctor**—After you've done your homework and you have a hunch based on solid research, talk to the doctor and share your findings. Bring appropriate documentation if you think it will be helpful, but don't inundate the doctor with information.

So where did I get all this information? In addition to my parent forums, I got it through the Internet, of course. Cyberspace had become my go-to tool for research, **but be warned**; it's also a great place to find *mis*information! I never let my online searches serve as my "final" answers, but more than once I found information that *did* relate to my son's case and was helpful to the doctors. The key is to utilize self-control and maintain balance. There are probably hundreds of web pages that will support whatever hypothesis you may have, or convince you that your child has X, Y, or Z according to the symptoms you've chosen to search, but more than likely, these diagnoses are inaccurate. Don't let yourself get sucked into that trap; it's counterproductive! It will drain you emotionally, as well as become a black hole absorbing all your time.

When searching the Internet, I made sure to look in reputable places, such as PubMed (a database of research published in reputable medical journals worldwide), the National Institutes of Health (NIH), and the Arthritis Foundation websites. I also limited the amount of time I spent on research. I steered clear of search engines, since they are not too picky about sources and can return some very odd, depressing, or skewed results. I used the reliable results to get some advance information that I could discuss *with* our doctors and be prepared for the things they might tell me. With the massive amounts of data out there, right at our fingertips (even from our phones), it can be hard to be disciplined in this area, but the benefits are worth it.

The Power of Sharing

In addition to focused and limited research, the Internet also helped me cope by providing an outlet to express my feelings and update others on my children's conditions. A few months into Grant's first chronic episode, I found that I was frequently drained from recounting the story and detailing his current ups, downs, and status to a number of well-meaning friends and family members. As much as I appreciated all of these folks being genuinely concerned and interested, repeating bad news over and over was taking a heavy toll on me. I might start the day with a good attitude, but after retelling the story for the fourth or fifth time, I would find myself on the verge of tears or in a funk that was hard to shake. I wanted to keep everyone informed, but it was killing me emotionally and it wasn't healthy. That's when I discovered blogging.

Blogging saved my sanity. I could sit down, write, review, revise, and let go … all before I hit the share button. I could recount some very emotional experiences and work through them, and I only had to relive it once. Grant was a pretty private person at the time, and at his request I made the blog private, by invitation only to our friends and family. Some days, so many things had happened that I would need to make multiple entries to keep everyone informed, particularly when he was in the hospital. Other times, we would hit glorious slow spots where there would be no medical updates for a few days, or even weeks. Recently, I have even gone up to a month without posting and have gotten a nudge from our readers for an update, even if it's just about what's going on in our "uneventful" life.

Blogging allowed me to share without draining myself emotionally. It permitted me to address the negative things happening in our lives at the moment, and then turn to more positive thinking the rest of the day. It freed up the time I was spending on the phone explaining our situation multiple times. Although this may seem small, it was very significant. Recounting our five-minute story ten times over the course of the day took almost an hour; time that I could have used to tie up loose ends in our everyday life or even take that warm bath I mentioned earlier. It insulated me from the irritation I would inevitably feel when our "big stuff" was trumped by the minor bumps that friends were facing in their proverbial road. Sometimes it's hard not to get grumpy when a friend asks if your child is out of his wheelchair yet, then goes on to say how awful it was for their kid when he twisted an ankle at soccer practice! (If they only knew how badly we wished *we* were at soccer practice, or that a twisted ankle was our biggest issue that day.) Telling our story in the blogosphere allowed me to avoid these situations and keep myself on a more even keel.

I still received positive wishes and feedback through comments on my blog, but I could read them when I was up to it. When I picked up the phone to talk to a friend, I could talk to them like a friend … they already knew about Grant (from checking the blog) and it took the pressure off for both sides. I could talk about meeting for coffee, since I now had a sliver of time! We could discuss the weather or the Kardashians or if I should get highlights or lowlights when I had my hair done next. It helped me make JA part of my life rather than the focus of our life, allowing me to regain a semblance of *my* normal life, and that was even better than a trip to Tahiti.

Finding Your Way Back to Normal

Many of the other JA parents with whom I have come into contact also find blogging helpful for many of the same reasons I mentioned. Not everyone is a blogger, though. However, even if you don't use social media, you can still use writing to reduce stress. Writing is a very powerful tool that can help you get back in touch with your emotions and work through feelings without getting sidetracked or clouded by another person's input, and you can do it without going public. When you write, you are alone with your thoughts. If you don't blog, then I would recommend keeping a journal. Many times I used my own blog as a journal and have been able to look back through the entries to remind myself how much we have been through and how far we have come.

It makes me happy all over again to read about some of our victories that may have been forgotten, or to recognize the cyclical nature of this disease, remembering that we have been through valleys before and a peak is around the corner. Personal journaling is a good complement to the medical journal we discussed earlier in the book. Sometimes looking at the medical journal in tandem with my blog posts around the same time has given me even more insight into my children's condition. I noticed that when I was down in the dumps that they were, too, and sometimes that even resulted in amplified pain and less restful sleep for *them*. Primarily, the blog did the most for me, but it did have other

STICKING TOGETHER by DANIELLE

Like many chronic illnesses, juvenile arthritis has its own community. Since my daughter Emily was diagnosed, I have formed lifelong relationships with other parents in the JA community—relationships that have helped my family and me not only learn more about this disease, but have also provided invaluable guidance and support. From the very beginning, I have leaned heavily on this resource.

During the week that Emily was diagnosed with dermatomyositis, I logged onto a family computer at the hospital. I wasn't expecting our first visit to this new doctor to last six days! Feeling lost, I began searching for some direction and found a group invite on my Facebook page, which led to a JA forum. Chatting with this group of JA moms in real time was like an epiphany. I realized that I wasn't alone, after all.

Another local mom suggested that I begin blogging. One thing led to another, and soon I began to "meet" other JA moms with the same questions and concerns I had, who were willing to share their experience. Thanks to one of my favorite Arthritis Foundation employees, I was introduced to another local online group. It was really neat to easily find people who lived close to each other. We started meeting up—sometimes by accident and sometimes at planned events.

More than just a source of information, one of the first moms I met online has become one of my dearest friends. We began communicating just after her son was diagnosed and over the years have shared both laughs and tears. Our kids have also become friends and often play together, along with other JA families. We have found that our children support each other in ways that their well friends cannot.

This friend and I have also both become proud advocates for juvenile arthritis, though, admittedly, she is more active in this role. At a recent Arthritis Foundation event, this particular mom and her son's team raised over $10,000! To top things off, her son even had his favorite professional baseball player come hang out with him at the event!

The bottom line is that knowing other JA families is very important. They intuitively understand the things *we* think about, worry about, and want other people to know. With them, you don't have to explain why you don't (or can't) make plans and why we always try to see the good in everything. Things are hard enough as it is. When friends and family just don't get it, having a JA family can make life a little easier.

benefits as well. This is why I hope you will take up some form of writing, even if it's just for yourself.

Some take writing even further and use it as a recognized form of therapy, through poetry, stories, or letters, or have expanded these feelings into visual art, similar to the art therapy programs that are so popular in the children's hospitals. Writing and art don't have a monopoly on the "processing feelings" market, though. There are many effective outlets for expressing your emotions. For instance, I have a couple friends who love to cook and swear that nothing releases pent-up stress like tenderizing meat with a mallet, getting elbow deep into kneading dough, or decorating a beautiful cake! For others, exercise may be their escape, pounding their stresses out on the pavement or willing it away through a quiet mind at yoga. Whatever it may be, it's important to find what works best for you and then do it. Take off a few of those hats every now and again, relax, recharge, and allow yourself to be YOU.

WRITING AS A RIGHTING JOURNEY by SUZANNE

I have had a few careers, including psychotherapist, movement educator, and landscape designer. During each of these vocations and throughout my life, I have kept journals, as well as written and published poetry. Writing was a constant in my life, and yet, when my daughter was diagnosed with juvenile myositis, a rare, autoimmune disease, at age six, I found I could not write.

For more than a year we'd searched for a diagnosis and I'd been writing the whole time. But once the actual illness was named, a new set of problems and feelings arose, and I was overwhelmed. After a few months, a friend and fellow poet sat me down and gave me a couple of writing exercises, which "broke the dam." I was released, and with a rush, the words, feelings, and thoughts came pouring out. I wrote about my experiences parenting a child with a chronic illness, one for which there is no cure (though there are treatments and, now, after five years, she is in remission).

Whatever came out on the page became poems, but these verses were not for others to read, at least not initially. This writing was for me and my sanity; for my health and well-being; to keep me a functioning, thinking advocate and parent. (I kept a separate blog/website to inform friends and family about my daughter's medical progress.) Eventually I took the poems to my writing group, and with their encouragement, I wrote and received grants to continue this poetic journey, and then to publish them.

Since then, I have continued to write and have tried to understand more about how the act of writing is a therapeutic function. Some brain research supports this idea. A simplified way to understand this concept is that our emotional brain center is located in the amygdala, which is where our instinctual, genetically programmed responses for flight or fight are triggered. These reactions then set off a whole set of unconscious bodily responses, raising levels of stress hormones and blood pressure, possibly overwhelming our capacities for calm and clear thinking. Our prefrontal cortex, which allows us to reflect on our emotions and to think more objectively, is simply not engaged at the same time as we are flooded by emotions in our amygdala. (LeDoux 2002)

The process of writing can allow a quieting of the amygdala and an engagement of the prefrontal cortex. But not all forms of writing actually do this. When I was being trained as a psychotherapist in the expressive arts, the prevailing thinking was to "get out" your feelings. That act of expression was a catharsis, and many experts thought that catharsis alone was sufficient to change people's actions and well-being. But what if writing about traumatic experiences simply reactivates the amygdala? In that case, expression doesn't help us move forward in our lives or contain those overwhelming and often unconscious feelings in a productive way.

Releasing feelings is only one step in the process. As an artist/poet, I had learned that raw, undigested feelings spat out onto a page did not a poem make. With some distance from the initial writing, I could go back and revise, finding better images or metaphors to "hold" the experiences and convey it to others. This revision (re-seeing) was also a thinking process. Though I didn't know it then, it probably was engaging my prefrontal cortex and allowing me to both experience the feelings and think about them.

This act of creation began to feel nurturing, like good, healthy food or a day at the beach. When I felt depleted as a caretaker, the act of writing poems or stories about my experience not only relieved stress and made me better able to advocate for my child because my thinking was clearer, it also gave me energy. It filled me like a hidden stream fills a newly dug well.

Over the past few years, I've begun teaching a writing workshop for parents who have children with ongoing health issues and have devised a framework for these classes based on many other people's ideas. I draw from brain researchers (Joseph LeDoux and Judy Willis), psychologists (Beth Jacobs, Ph.D.), and writing teachers and poets (John Fox and Louise DeSalvo). I call my work *Writing as a Righting Journey*. I incorporate exercises that encourage releasing/expressing feelings about our current situations, and then follow them with refocusing exercises that help us move into thinking about those feelings or situations and provide ways to contain and refocus our awareness. Then we put those ideas into a creative form of writing using metaphors and images, sound and simile—all the tools of creative writing—to help move people into the realm of gaining some joy or energetic rejuvenation, grounding our emotion with the capacity to think and communicate to others.

I think this last piece—communicating with others—is important. Though we may not choose to share our writing, when we do, we also close the loop on isolation. The act of creation is a powerful and healing one. When we put our creations out into the world we build bridges to others; we build community; we renew ourselves and bring a measure of hope to our situations and, possibly, to others. It's one way to make meaning out of a difficult situation.

CHAPTER THIRTEEN

Playing It Day by Day

Sometimes people ask me what our day-to-day life has been like since our boys were diagnosed with JA. It's not an easy question to answer, because there is no typical day. Our life has changed and continues to evolve. Having a family member with a serious chronic illness makes life unpredictable and uncertain. With many other health issues, such as a broken bone or an appendectomy, for example, the worst presents itself and then gradually gets better through rest, medications, therapies, and time. Chronic illnesses such as JA are more like a roller-coaster ride, with ups and downs, and little to no warning as to which way the track will turn. Although we can hope for remission, there is no cure. JA is a permanent part of our life, and therefore we must recognize it and adjust accordingly. Over time, we have come to realize that we can be our happiest if we accept this new reality and make the most of every day—within the context of that particular day. Let me explain …

Learn to Go with the Flow

Control is an issue that plagues many JA parents. Before having a "sick" kid, many parents enjoy exercising a fair amount of control over their own lives and the lives of their children. Parents work, kids go to school, and what to do in our leisure time is usually decided by interests and financial feasibility. A typical day in a "normal" family might consist of waking at a set time, going to school, grabbing a snack before soccer practice, doing some homework, eating dinner, watching a little TV, and then complying with a set bedtime. *All* of these activities are *variables* when dealing with JA. If the child had a difficult night, then waking up early to get to school may be counterproductive. If chicken pox or the flu is making rounds at school, even a "good" day may need to be spent at home, rather than risking exposure and making the situation worse. If JA is starting to flare, soccer practice might be out, and dinnertime may need to be adjusted to accommodate the next round of meds. For instance, if a particular medication needs to be taken on an empty stomach and is due at six o'clock, then dinner has to be moved two hours earlier or later. Homework could be tabled due to brain fog or an earlier bedtime to make up for the lack of sleep from the previous night (unless, of course, meds are due later than bedtime, which means you are up even longer). You get the idea—the possible "ifs" are endless.

A chronic illness can turn everything upside down. Your routine becomes defined by the illness and its whims, rather than the plans you made or the intentions you had! For many, this is one of the hardest pills to swallow. To add to the frustration, all the other conditions that normally determine whether or not an activity happens can be met—you have the time, interest, desire, and funds—but with JA, the physical ability to comply is the deciding factor, and that can change at the drop of a hat. Initially, the inability to do the things we wanted to do made me very sad. I mourned the lost opportunities for my kids—the parties and sleepovers they missed, the ball games they didn't play, the vacations we never took, especially if we had them planned and then had to cancel.

Later, when Grant started getting better, the insecurity drove me batty. I hated not knowing when we could count on doing something, or being disappointed when we had to cancel because the situation had changed, *again*. And then it dawned on me, the only way to regain control was to let it go and embrace going with the flow. I learned that the changes that come along with JA could work both ways—sometimes preventing us from doing what we wanted, but other times when we thought we would be unable to do something, we were pleasantly surprised with a turn for the better! Every day became a new adventure, a different opportunity, and a fresh start.

I started looking at things from an entirely new perspective, from the vantage point of our "new normal." Even on the days when things were not going very well, I could control what happened within the circumstances we were given *that* day. Instead of wasting time and energy being disappointed, we could make the best of the situation—we could spend the day catching up and doing a jigsaw puzzle or having a James Bond movie marathon. We simply made a different kind of fun. If we were having a particularly good day, we scrambled to make plans to take advantage of it, instead of putting things off until later. We began to embrace the philosophy of carpe diem—or seize the day.

Discover the Silver Lining

I know you've heard it said many times—there is a silver lining in every rain cloud—but it's true. We have found a positive side to JA; it has taught us to live life a little more fully, appreciating even the smallest victories and the simplest of pleasures. It has given me a different perspective and, subsequently, I have taught my kids to embrace the moment in the same way. This doesn't mean we never make plans, but rather that we've learned not to be too disappointed if we have to cancel, reschedule, or revise those plans. We have also found that a missed opportunity in one area often turns into a completely unexpected (and sometimes delightful) prospect that we never would have experienced otherwise. We are more flexible, with a plan A, B, and C, just in case things don't go exactly as we hoped. We have learned to keep our plans whenever possible, but also to modify them in a realistic (and enjoyable) way when necessary. And on the other side, when we've been able to do things we didn't think we could after an unexpected improvement, we've come to appreciate it all the more. If everyone is having a good (or great) day, we don't let that go to waste—we're out there taking advantage of every opportunity. As a result, a whole new world has opened up to us, one that we never had the ability to see before.

THE BuCKET LIST

It doesn't seem right that my 11-year-old came to me with the idea of developing a bucket list. I asked him if he really knew what a "bucket list" meant. He did. He had overheard a couple medical residents discussing his case at the hospital and, for the first time, recognized how fragile his life could be. There were so many things he wanted to do that he hadn't done yet, and he realized that he might not have forever to do them.

While that's true for all of us, many adults go through life without coming to this realization—until they hit their midlife crisis. Yet here was my sixth grader planning his days with his own mortality in mind. It was a real eye opener.

At first, I didn't encourage the list. To be honest, I thought it was a bit morbid. I knew he would pull through, even though we had just experienced a very scary time. But, then I reconsidered. Grant's list included very realistic attainable goals, sprinkled with a few dreams. Putting them on paper was powerful! It gave him motivation to get out of that hospital bed and start moving as soon as he could, because he no longer took time for granted.

As he started to get better, we knocked as many of the easy things as we could off the list. Some goals were simple and sweet, like earning enough money (on his own) to buy me a birthday gift, getting a straight A report card, and hitting a home run. Other items were a little more ambitious, such as catching a 100-pound fish, visiting Peru, and raising ten thousand dollars for charity on his own! Most of his wishes fell somewhere in between, like visiting all 50 states and every major league stadium/arena, or eating at the Travel Channel's *101 Chowdown Countdown* restaurants.

Reading through his list surprised me in places and was totally predictable in others, but it had a profound effect on me. Grant's list made me realize that I had the ability to help him through this difficult time in his life by helping him give it more meaning. As we worked our way through the list, there was a sense of accomplishment with every checkmark. He took batting lessons and made his first home run. He got straight As. He shoveled the neighbors' driveways and bought me noise-cancelling headphones. He set up a FirstGiving web page for charity. Even when he wasn't physically able to achieve some of his goals, he could still research them or lay the groundwork to make things happen later. For instance, he wrote a 30-page essay about Peru, so if we get the chance to travel there, we know all about the history, culture, and where to go.

Instead of focusing on his illness and waiting for the other shoe to drop, he began to anticipate the future. He was excited again. If he felt well enough and could find a good deal, we would pick up last-minute tickets to the closest sporting event and cross another stadium off the list. On one occasion, as we were passing through Denver visiting friends, we found tickets to a Colorado Rockies' game for just *one* dollar! Even though Grant wasn't feeling well enough to stay for the entire game, we got out for a bit, and he had the satisfaction of making another checkmark. We started taking advantage of every opportunity and using it to the best of our abilities.

But it wasn't just Grant who benefited from the bucket list: We all started to follow his lead. We began looking at life a little differently. Although I still had many responsibilities to take care of each day, when I finished with those tasks I began to ask myself "What can *I* do to live? … to enjoy my life? … to not take this day for granted?" The bucket list did more than crystallize long- and short-term goals or put a few dreams on paper: It pushed us to *do* things, instead of just thinking about them.

Three and a half years later, Grant has crossed off nearly half of the items on his original list, but it continues to evolve. He has added more goals and deleted a few items that aren't such a big deal anymore. He is studying German on his own so he'll be prepared for a trip to Europe (specifically Germany and Switzerland) if the opportunity arises. Before we travel, he determines if any *Chowdown* restaurants are in the area so we can stop in for a bite. He has learned to make the most of every day and every opportunity, regardless of the circumstances. He has learned to plan, as well as to act. The bucket list that I was originally skeptical of has played an integral role in making him a whole child again and enriched our lives in the process.

When your child is very ill, it's not difficult to live your life one day at a time. When things are bad, the world sort of stops and you just concentrate on getting your child better. Each day is focused on making some progress and getting back to normal. When your child is doing well, it's also fairly easy. Adjustments are usually small when your child is in a good place, and it doesn't take as much effort to keep things moving along smoothly. For us, the hardest times have been those in-between phases that make up the bulk of your life when your child is not yet in remission. These are the times when the doctors are figuring out the right treatment plan, and you have to adjust to medication changes. Or the times you must deal with a completely unexpected flare, or a regular childhood illness on top of JA. It's the difficultly of experiencing a "down" when you thought you were heading "up." These are the times when you must learn to thrive within, if you want to make the most of your life and help your child live in a happier place.

The Spoon Theory

As you plan your day, the first thing you have to consider is your child's threshold for activity. There is a great anecdote written by Christine Miserandino entitled "The Spoon Theory" that illustrates this point beautifully. Picture yourself being handed a fistful of spoons. Each spoon represents the ability to do an activity, like a type of currency. If you want to do something, it will cost you a spoon. When all the spoons are gone, that's it. You don't have anything left to "spend" on more activities. When your child is experiencing an acute episode, it may take all their "spoons" just to get out of bed, shower, dress, and eat breakfast. If they spend them too fast or on the wrong things, there won't be any left. You have to choose carefully, because when they're gone, they're gone!

I would like to take Miserando's analogy one step further: when your child is doing well, his or her spoons might be worth more. The same number of spoons may get you more mileage on a different day. Your child may need two or three to go to school, a couple more to do his homework and spend some time with friends, and may even have one left over at the end of the day. You have to figure out the exchange rate for the day, based on your child's current condition. When you know how many spoons you have for the day, and you also know what the current exchange rate will be, then you can determine what is within the realm of possibility for that day and how you can maximize its potential.

A few days after Grant got out of the hospital the first time, he was weak and still pretty sick, but he was also tired of spending so much time inside after days at the hospital followed by days in his room. I knew he was getting stir crazy, but even walking to the car for a doctor's appointment was exhausting. I wasn't sure what I could do to meet his needs, while still being a responsible parent. What he really needed was a day out, but he didn't have much in him to make that happen, so we came up with a creative solution. We rented a wheelchair, and I pushed him along the outdoor trails of the botanical garden near our home. He was happy to be outside, and we both enjoyed the fresh air and change of scenery, but the trip was not overtaxing.

A few weeks later, when Grant was feeling better, we went to the arboretum with his brother. He was feeling well enough to play at the playground for a very short time, but the half-mile walk to the playground *and* using the equipment would have been too much for him. So, we used the wheelchair to get him to the site, and despite the strange looks we got when he hopped out to play, that 15 minutes of being "normal" really lifted his spirits. Using the wheelchair for the least important part of the outing enabled him to enjoy an element of his life he had been missing.

In the same vein, Grant learned to modify his social outings into manageable portions. During his seventh grade year, he was invited to many Bar and Bat Mitzvahs. Although he was going to school three to four days a week at the time, he still didn't have the stamina to attend the full duration of these religious services and parties. Depending on how he was feeling, I would allow him to take the group transportation along with his friends, and then I would pick him up after an hour or two, giving him time to make an appearance and socialize some, but before he was too worn out or miserable. As he continued to improve, he would let his friends know that he was up for a round of Frisbee golf, but a game of flag football might be too much for him. We tailored his activities and activity levels to the number of spoons we knew he had—but we didn't allow him to use JA as an excuse not to keep living his life.

Find the Right Balance

The second thing you must consider is balance. Over the last few years, Grant hasn't had the ability to keep up with all the same activities and expectations of the average kid. In the beginning, our ups and downs came rather unpredictably. Although we still have them, it seems as though the bad times are not as severe, and the good times stay around much longer. We still suffer through the same cycles, but we have more time to catch our breath. Even though Grant isn't in remission yet, and there is no cure, there is still hope. We appreciate the longer periods of respite and are a little stronger when we deal with the setbacks. We have modified *all* areas of his life so that the expectations are realistic. If he has enough spoons to attend school but not to do anything else, then school needs to be modified at that time. We have made a point to ensure he has enough spoons to create a good mix of real-life activities, including school, chores, *and* fun, just like other kids. We make sure there is enough time and energy left over (even if we have to cut back on his responsibilities a little) so he can still enjoy his life, although we encourage him to use the bulk of his spoons to function like his peers.

In time, we have found that accepting this new reality and making the most of it, rather than being disgruntled about what we can't do, have allowed us to be much happier. It has challenged us to think of new and creative things to do with our time and made us more prepared to seize the day, regardless of what that day might bring. Playing it day-by-day with an eye on the future has given us a peace that I'm not sure we had even before our children had a chronic illness. We've made JA work *for* us, instead of against us.

CHAPTER FOURTEEN

Getting Involved

There are plenty of ways to become involved with the JA community; you can choose to do a little or a lot—whatever works for you. Initially, you can utilize the activities and resources offered by various foundations and organizations to get connected with others in your situation. JA activities are constructed to provide safe, physically possible enrichment experiences for you and your family despite the possible limitations of the illness. Alternatively, the resources offered by these groups can serve as a means to further the cause for research, legislation, and education that will affect others suffering from this disease. There are always opportunities to learn from and participate in these offerings. What you do, and how you do it, is up to you.

Camps, Conferences, and Other Fun Stuff

For many families, the first step is just becoming acquainted with the organizations that deal with their diagnosis. Many of these organizations offer camps, conventions, seminars, family fun days, or social events to bring families together and educate participants about their condition. Getting a feel for these services and participating in some of their offerings will also help you decide which groups are a good fit if you should decide to volunteer or donate resources.

Getting involved with other families and allowing your children to make connections with other kids like them are very important parts of dealing with their diagnosis. Not only do they serve as a means of increasing your understanding and education about various aspects of the disease, they allow you to share your experiences and possibly help other families. Organized events can provide valuable information and guidance for volunteer opportunities, as well.

While visiting family in Florida, my kids and I were lucky enough to participate in one of the Arthritis Foundation (AF) family days at the local museum of science and industry. Like many of these offerings, the event was free to preregistered families. The day started with a program highlighting advances made in research and medications, followed by a question-and-answer session. They also outlined ways for families to get involved, especially in the upcoming Arthritis Walk. After the short program, the kids were allowed to mingle with each other and explore the museum. Participants were identified by stickers worn on their shirts, which made it easy to find other JA families and strike up a conversation as we explored the exhibits on our own time. We even had a chance to meet some of our online friends from the JA forums. We came away from this event a little more educated and a lot more connected, while enjoying a fun outing with kids just like ours.

Although we have yet to participate in a camp, many of our JA family friends have had positive experiences. And, camps are not just for kids! Although there are many youth camp offerings that specifically deal with JA, there are also camps and retreat weekends for JA families that focus on the *entire* family. The Serious Fun camps, which were founded by Paul Newman and include the Painted Turtle near Los Angeles, Camp Boggy Creek in Florida, and others, have specific weeks/weekends dedicated to different medical conditions, as well as a number of family programs. Most local chapters of the Arthritis Foundation have youth or family camp programs as well.

Mixing Business and Pleasure

While some events are focused on play, others have a bigger volunteer or work component. That doesn't mean they still can't be fun though! In March of 2013, we connected with other families and advocates from around the nation while attending a three-day summit presented by the National Arthritis Foundation. In addition to informative programs about arthritis, we were able to learn about pending legislation that could affect the 300,000 children and 50 million adults living with arthritis in the United States. The advocacy summit educated, but it also gave us a chance to meet, face-to-face, with senators, congressmen, and their staff members in Washington, D.C., to highlight legislation important to our cause. Volunteering to travel and attend a multiday conference or summit is a big commitment, but in our case, it was an opportunity to make a large impact in very little time. We made great connections, learned quite a bit, and made an impression on our elected officials.

The Arthritis Advocacy Summit is not the only way to make an impact. Many summit attendees, including myself, are also "Arthritis Ambassadors" for the Arthritis Foundation. Arthritis Ambassadors commit to participating for one hour each month, alternating between listening in on a conference call and executing a "call to action." For a commitment of only 12 hours a year, these volunteers perform assignments such as writing press releases for their local media and calling their congressperson, highlighting issues important to arthritis sufferers across the country.

The American Autoimmune Related Disease Association (AARDA) provides another opportunity to pursue advocacy activities and applies a broader scope than "just" arthritis. Since many children with JA can also have overlapping autoimmune diseases, the AARDA provides a wealth of information for families who suffer from related conditions, as well as the opportunity to help through organized or "virtual walks" that do not have a preset time or place.

These are just a couple examples of "work" that can benefit the cause. There are a multitude of volunteer opportunities—from lobbying and fundraising, to working a concession stand or registration table at an event—the opportunities are as varied as the people who commit to helping. For any skill or interest you might possess, there is a volunteer opportunity to match it, especially within large organizations. You might man a phone bank for call-in donations, serve as a board member, give a speech, paint an office, design a brochure, or have a garage sale. The possibilities to contribute are endless.

Taking It One Step Further—Parents on a Mission

As great as many of these foundations and organizations are, you may be drawn to a particular mission they don't include. If established organizations don't address a certain need, *you* can be the one to make the difference! For example, although the Arthritis Foundation does a tremendous job promoting *all* forms of arthritis, some parents felt it would be beneficial to create a charitable organization that focused *only* on JA; thus the Juvenile Arthritis Association (JAA) was born.

The JAA began as the brainchild of parents Joel Rothman and Laura Schultz, who formed the group to increase awareness and funding specifically for pediatric rheumatologic diseases. While juvenile arthritis affects approximately one in every 250 children, the estimated level of private funding for JA hovers around two million dollars annually. Compare this to the incidence of juvenile diabetes, which affects approximately one in 500 children, but receives nearly *two hundred million* dollars in private funding annually. With statistics like these, the need for a specific JA oriented group is plain. These parents recognized a need and filled it. Even in its first year, the JAA recruited a number of dedicated volunteers and spokespeople, while hosting exciting events such as a Hollywood celebrity yard sale, proving that the "big guys" aren't the only ones who can successfully execute a vision.

Prior to the founding of the JAA, another small group of parents banded together to provide support for one of the very specific under-represented diseases under the JA umbrella: juvenile myositis (JM). Cure JM was founded in 2003 by Harriet Bollar, Shari Hume, and Lisa Felix.

It started simply as a grassroots effort to provide support for families and raise funds to find a cure. Their first endeavor was a modest lemonade stand, but they have grown substantially over the last decade, raising more than four million dollars to date, assisting in the development of two research centers, and funding *Myositis and You*, a book written by more than 100 doctors and the first reference guide to be published about JM. What started as the idea of a couple moms and one grandparent has become a significant resource within the JM community.

Another example of a parent taking matters into her own hands is an organization called Stop CAID Now!, which focuses on childhood auto-inflammatory diseases. It began as the dream of one mom and has become an internationally recognized voice for children with any form of autoimmune or auto-inflammatory disease. As the parent of a child with this type of rare disease and frustrated by the inability to get help for her child, Lisa Moreno Dickinson decided to take action. She recognized the need to include many rare AI/AIF conditions as one voice, since each illness in isolation affected such a small number of children. Utilizing resources from interests across a number of conditions has allowed Stop CAID Now! to be strengthened by numbers and fulfill their mission of educating medical professionals about these diseases, resulting in earlier diagnosis and focused treatments for many serious but rare illnesses. Stop CAID Now! has also been instrumental in the development of the very first CAID clinic at the Cleveland Clinic Children's Hospital in Ohio, as well as the publication of a book that helps kids understand their illness.

Although different in scope and focus, these three organizations have one thing in common: they were developed by parents who wanted to target a specific cause that previously received just a portion of attention within a broader charity. By developing a nonprofit with a single focus, they were able to garner additional awareness and resources for the conditions that affected their children the most, while helping countless others.

The Juvenile Arthritis Association, CureJM, and Stop CAID Now! were founded to highlight and support specific diagnoses under the general arthritis umbrella. Although they began as grassroots efforts, each has gained a national presence. On a completely different note, when

Rochelle Lentini and Dawn Veselka started their High-5-Club, they decided to keep things local. Each has children with chronic rheumatic illnesses that caused them to spend time in the hospital, both as inpatients on the ward and outpatients in the infusion center. By noticing what was going on around them, these moms realized they could make a huge difference in the lives of the children and families who were crossing their paths. While children with some conditions were recognized for completing procedures with bravery, children with other conditions were not, even though they were undergoing the same exact treatments! They also recognized that some of these same families were going without food, treatments, or therapies in order to afford other parts of their medical care. The High-5-Club reaches out to these families to level the playing field, assist those who need it most, and recognize *all* kids with chronic illness for their bravery. Although they were inspired by the issues faced by JA families, their charity has filled a need that relates to many conditions, including JA.

Taking things one step further is not just about developing new 501c3 (nonprofit) organizations, however. Sometimes our unique experiences and perspectives can provide insight for the development of a new product or service that would benefit the JA community. Getting involved can mean recognizing a need and developing a product to fill it, thereby improving the lives of others. Jennifer Leone, another JM mom, wanted to give her daughter more freedom—a difficult dilemma with a strict medication schedule. In order to allow her uninterrupted access to ballet training without altering her medication schedule, Jennifer began taping her daughter's medications to her reusable water bottle. Then the idea struck. She developed and patented a product called the Pillid that safely secures medications between the water bottle and its cap. Several Pillids can be stacked to include keys, cash, or other small sundries. It was a simple concept that gave her daughter back her independence, and she began to produce and promote them so others could experience the same freedom. Even though Pillid is a commercial enterprise, this type of product fills a unique niche for chronically ill children and adults, and a portion of the proceeds are contributed to Cure JM.

Each of these worthwhile organizations was founded by regular parents, just like you and me. They recognized a need, found their niche, and created a groundbreaking way to get involved.

Kids Get Involved, Too!

Adults don't have a monopoly on great ideas or charitable contributions. Getting involved can include getting your *kids* involved, and not just with JA related activities. It's easy to include your children on the annual AF Jingle Bell Run or in a family fun day event. They can speak at events or be an event honoree. They can participate and volunteer in many capacities, just like adults; but they can also bring attention to JA in their own special way.

Kaci Taylor knows how difficult life can be with an autoimmune disease. She has watched for years while her younger sister Kory traveled to the hospital for infusions and treatments. Being in the hospital is no fun, even as an outpatient, so Kaci decided to do something to make things just a little better. As a high school freshman, she developed a website (www.kacitaylor.me) and mission statement, providing fun fleece blankets or "cozies" to hurricane victims, the local women's shelter, and, of course, to children in the hospital who could use the extra cheer. Currently, she will ship a cozie anywhere, to anyone in need, or anyone who needs to feel loved and appreciated. Even as a young adult, Kaci is making a positive impact and getting involved in a way that speaks to her, being familiar with the happiness that a gift of comfort can bring to a child in the hospital, and taking it one step further to help many others.

My younger son Evan has volunteered for many 5-K charity runs, lobbied at the Capitol, and participated in family fun days. His real love, however, is animals. During one of his brother's hospital visits in Los Angeles, he happened to peek over my shoulder to see a very sad post on my social media. It was a plea for help from one of my local friends. That day several puppies in Irving, Texas, were scheduled to be euthanized due to overcrowding … beautiful, healthy young dogs whose eyes touched his soul. Evan was beside himself. He pledged all his

Christmas money in order to give them a chance (animal rescues will sometimes save a dog that has some funding). He asked me to e-mail the shelter, call friends, and other rescue groups. Meanwhile, he started e-mailing everyone *he* could. One of the e-mails made it through to the shelter director, who was moved by our story. She shared the story with a local rescue organization, which then pulled the remaining four animals, so that all 14 dogs originally scheduled for euthanasia were spared.

But he didn't stop there. When we were coming back through Texas, he visited the remaining dogs that had been moved to the Humane Society (a no-kill shelter), and he agreed to help with publicity. As the story traveled, volunteers sent us messages with renewed hope for their very emotional and often sad jobs. We helped transport a dog to its new owners and found a home to permanently place another. We 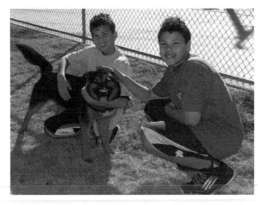 even took on two foster dogs ourselves. In addition, we developed a friendship with the original rescue organization. Evan's enthusiasm spread to Grant and the rest of our family.

So how does this relate to getting involved with JA? It has come full circle. Evan and Grant are now known among many of the shelter volunteers and online support community for Irving animals. Many had never heard of JA and were moved by children with their own issues working so hard for animal welfare. Several made pledges to Grant's web page, First-Giving (raising funds for Cure JM) or asked how *they* could help. In addition to raising awareness for the shelter, the rescue organization, the Humane Society, *and* their illness, another idea was brought to fruition. The rescue organization we originally worked with to save the "final four" developed a new 501c3 called Canine Compassionate Companions, which gives temperament-tested shelter animals a chance to be companions for the chronically ill or elderly, while assisting recipients with the cost and/or care associated with the ownership of a pet. They are currently working on training some of the dogs in the program to serve as "semi-assistance" dogs that can perform specific tasks for those who suffer from mild disabilities, but do not need or qualify for a certified service animal. Learning more about JA from this personal connection helped identify this need and marry it with another seemingly unrelated mission: to save shelter animals.

Medical Studies, Drug Trials, and Registries

Another way to advance research and treatment options is through medical studies and drug trials. Although many people may not think about these options as a way to get involved, they're a very important part of developing new treatments and better understanding of the diseases with which our children live.

Medical studies focus on proving a hypothesis for research purposes. They may or may not include the administration of medications. A few years ago, our family participated in two studies related to pediatric pain. As a rheumatology patient, Grant was a chronic pain sufferer. While we were visiting our team at UCLA, we were made aware of a few studies in which Grant was qualified to participate. One study involved the observation and recording of responses to a mild pain stimulus across different members of the same family. Another study looked at the impact of peer mentorship in the management of pain symptoms in adolescents. When given the opportunity, Grant was eager to participate since his inclusion might result in helping other kids, with absolutely no personal risk. Our part in the first study only took a few hours, and the other study was completed in about two months via periodic phone conversations with his peer mentor group.

Other studies can be more extensive, such as the Study of Families with Twins or Siblings Discordant for Rheumatic Disorders at the National Institutes of Health in Washington, D.C. Several of our friends have been involved with this study that looks at twins or same gender siblings less than one year apart where only one child has a rheumatic condition. Both siblings undergo an extensive review of medical history, physical exam, and lab work in order to discover clues as to why some children may be more disposed than others to the development of these diseases.

To find out about trials that your family may be eligible to participate in, you can visit www.clinicaltrials.gov and enter key words that correspond with your specific condition. Trials that match your criteria will be listed, along with the locations that are participating in recruitment and data collection. Alternatively, your rheumatologist or other specialist may recommend a particular study for which your child is a particularly good candidate. Although many studies are operated strictly on a volunteer basis, others may provide a small stipend or pay for expenses related to your participation. As with any other activity, it's important to research the program prior to your involvement to determine if the study is right for you and if you are agreeable to the procedures associated with the study. In our case, Grant and Evan were both willing and eager to participate in research that could improve the lives of other children, especially if they included minimal or noninvasive procedures.

Similar to research studies, drug trials offer the opportunity to participate in research associated with drugs that are (1) not yet FDA approved, (2) not yet approved for use in pediatric patients, or (3) approved for a different condition, but being tested for effectiveness in an alternate use. Participation in drug trials can be a touchy subject with some parents. I have heard many differing opinions from "I would never use my child as a guinea pig" to "We were so desperate for help we would try anything," and many responses in between. There are many motivating factors, and they are unique to each family. Before any decision is made, several factors need to be considered:

- **Commitment**—Everyone needs to be onboard, including the child, especially if they are old enough to make solid cognitive decisions. Trying a new drug without FDA approval or research to back it can be a scary decision. You are in uncharted waters, so to speak, and outcomes cannot be guaranteed. Both parents (and an older child) should be aware of the possible risks and benefits associated with their participation.

- **Ramifications**—In addition to possible side effects or unforeseen issues, participating in a drug study *may* affect current treatments. For many drugs, there is a wash-out period, where other treatments that your child takes must be discontinued and cleared from his system, so as not to taint the results of the trial. Remember, the purpose of a drug trial is to test the effectiveness of an unproven drug, so the use of other medications that would cloud the picture must be discontinued. If the child is one of the participants who receives a placebo (that is, they believe they receive the drug, but are selected to take an inert substance instead), then their condition could be untreated for the duration of the trial.
- **Insurance**—It's critical that you check with your insurer prior to any involvement in a drug study. Carriers differ in their policies, so it's important to check if participation will result in the denial of future medical claims. Make sure you have proof of coverage for any medical issues that may arise as a result of the study, an agreement from the group executing the study to handle medical claims arising from it, or be prepared to handle those claims on your own if necessary.
- **Costs**—In addition to potential medical claims not covered by insurance, there may be costs associated with participating in a drug trial, including time off work and school or transportation. Some trials will provide funding to offset costs if you are accepted into the study.

After these factors are addressed, if the family still wants to move forward, it's time to enter the research phase. The first place to start is with your physician. Make sure he or she feels this would be an appropriate step in the care and treatment of your child, or at minimum have the reasonable expectation that it would do no harm. The next step is to conduct your own research using key terms on scholarly, well-respected Internet sites, such as Google Scholar, the NIH, or PubMed, to find out as much as you can about the drug and its possible side effects. Some questions you might want to ask are: "Is the drug approved for children in other countries, and if so, for how long?" "How many years has this drug been studied (in adults and in children)?" and "Have the side effects been minimal (or bearable) in the original application?"

Many drugs that were developed for one purpose have been found to have valuable off-label uses; that is, they are approved to treat some conditions and considered "safe," but not FDA approved to treat other illnesses. Some drug trials are used to approve drugs for these alternate purposes. Knowing the answers to the questions I've listed may encourage you to participate or sway your decision away from joining the trial.

If you are interested in finding available drug trials, your specialist can be instrumental in recommending the right study. To search on your own, the National Institutes of Health (NIH) and National Institute of Arthritis and Musculoskeletal and Skin Diseases (NIAMS) offer information on past, future, and current trials and studies.

In addition, participating in a patient registry can facilitate the process of finding the right study or trial. The Childhood Arthritis and Rheumatology Research Alliance (CARRA) provides several opportunities to get involved, including a patient registry. Friends of CARRA, the volunteer affiliate, helps to generate funds for future research studies, raises awareness about the activities of the organization, and promotes patient involvement in the ongoing studies undertaken by researchers and nearly 250 pediatric rheumatologists across the United States and Canada. They are an excellent resource for all conditions that fall under the JA umbrella.

From large foundations to parents and even children, getting involved can make a difference for JA, as well as the greater good. Everyone can play a role, and the types of roles are endless. I have only scratched the surface on the ways that you and your family might find to become involved and make a difference. Whatever direction you may choose, I hope you find the right niche for you *and* your children. The satisfaction and pride we have felt from getting involved has also been a gift to us! We've been privileged to connect, assist, and participate in many of these unique opportunities, helping our own family while helping others. (To get started, please see the Resources section for a list of organizations and websites.)

THE HIGH-5-CLUB by DAWN AND ROCHELLE

Spending hours every other week in a hospital infusion room can easily lead to feelings of despair and discouragement for the entire family dealing with chronic illness. As parents, our job is to teach our brave warriors how to combat the battle inside their body and cope with the mixed emotions. How do we empower these children who have lost so much control in their lives? By taking action.

Where there are problems, there are also solutions. Our kids, along with many of the other children receiving treatment, noticed that the treasure chest in the doctor's office lacked "value." These kids cope with a great deal, and the rewards being offered were definitely not worth the pain and suffering they endured. So, our children came up with a brilliant idea: for their birthdays they decided to host a great big birthday party where they would collect "treasures" instead of birthday presents, which gave all their friends an opportunity to get involved. The treasures that were donated not only brought smiles to the patients, but also filled our children and their friends with great pride and joy.

Later, we heard about families struggling with basic needs; having to choose between food for the week and gas to get their child to treatment. In our eyes, these choices were unacceptable. This problem also needed a solution. So, along with our children, we organized a food drive. But this was just the beginning, as the generosity and enthusiasm of our kids inspired us to do more.

Regular visits to the infusion room made us realize that the issue ran deeper than just prizes. Most people don't realize that, in a hospital setting, children with chronic illnesses receive infusions in a large open room alongside children with other illnesses such as cancer, hemophilia, gastrointestinal diseases, and multiple autoimmune conditions. There are many positive aspects to this arrangement, but it can be difficult for children with chronic illnesses to witness "end-of-treatment cele-brations," while their treatment is never-ending. Organizations that support childhood cancer have recognized the importance of celebrating milestones during treatment, along with the bravery that comes with enduring multiple frightening and invasive procedures. There are even national programs that recognize these achievements, and when children receive their final treatment there is usually a party in the infusion room. All these festivities take place in proximity to the multiple children who are sharing the same room ... all of whom are hoping for a cure.

When families and their children with chronic illnesses observe such celebrations, they struggle between feeling happy for the children who are rewarded or finished and feeling discouraged and frustrated knowing they may never have a similar celebration. When our own children asked, "When will I have my end-of-treatment celebration?" we were unable to answer them. This felt like another problem, so we began to think of ways to uplift and encourage *all* children with chronic illness.

It was becoming obvious to us that there was a wide variety of needs and many people who wanted to help, including friends and family who were constantly looking for quick and easy ways to support us. We found that people want to help but often don't know how. It was never our in-tention to start a nonprofit organization, but what started out as looking for little ways to lend a hand and empower our children has grown into the High-5-Club. We believe that every child deserves a "high five." The act of giving and receiving a high five is a universal gesture of encouragement and perseverance. It's a physical and social connection that delivers the message "you are not alone."

In developing this organization, we tried to widen our view and take in what others were sharing with us. By talking with other families, doctors, nurses, child life specialists, and social workers, as well as our family and friends, we identified the top needs in our community. Based on those needs, the High-5-Club has five core goals: (1) to assist families by offsetting the cost of treatments with food/gas/transportation gift cards; (2) to develop a website with resources for families; (3) to encourage and empower children with chronic illness by giving them a platform to encourage and help others; (4) to fund fellowships to offset the shortage of pediatric rheumatologists across the country; and (5) to provide micro-grants to fund alternative treatments not covered by insurance.

We encourage families to pause and look beyond their own needs and struggles as they endure treatments, therapies, and medical appointments. Our children have taught us that we can all reach out and make a difference in our own community—and in our own lives. It's inspirational to see the renewed sense of purpose that being a part of the High-5-Club has given our own children. They are so proud, and we are proud of them. Making these random acts of kindness benefits those on *both* sides in *big* ways!

(If you are interested in learning more about the High-5-Club and how you can encourage a child, please visit our website at www. high-5-club.org)

Resources

Blogs

Blogger and WordPress—two popular free blog hosting sites
www.blogger.com
wordpress.org
CaringBridge—online health support community and medical
blog hosting
www.caringbridge.org

Books

*Conquering Your Child's Chronic Pain: A Pediatrician's Guide for
Reclaiming a Normal Childhood*, by Lonnie K. Zeltzer and
Christina Blackett Schlank, William Morrow Paperbacks, 2005.
It's Not Just Growing Pains, by Thomas J.A. Lehman, M.D.,
Oxford University Press, USA, 2004.

Burnout in Children

www.elrophe.org/parenting-and-family-articles/24-children
-and-burnout
well.blogs.nytimes.com/2010/01/27/burned-out-so-are-your-kids/
www.sheknows.com/parenting/articles/2324/warning-signs
-of-stress-and-burnout-are-your-kids-doing-too-much

Camps

Serious Fun Network (founded by Paul Newman)
www.seriousfunnetwork.org
The Arthritis Foundation (access the main website, then search according to your state)
www.arthritis.org
In Europe www.otw.org.uk

Charitable Organizations/Projects

Canine Compassionate Companions
www.caninecompassionatecompanions.org
Cozies by Kaci
www.kacitaylor.me/KaciTaylor/Welcome.html
Dallas Fort-Worth Humane Society
dfwhumane.com
FirstGiving—online fundraising for your favorite charity
www.firstgiving.com/
Sample page: Grant Miller's FirstGiving page for Cure JM
(the page he set up to help others as part of his bucket list)
www.firstgiving.com/fundraiser/grant-miller/grantwmiller
High-5-Club
high-5-club.org
Irving Animal Shelter & Volunteer Support Organizations
www.cityofirving.org/animal-services/Animals
www.facebook.com/IrvingAnimalShelter
www.facebook.com/PawsForIrvingAnimals

Complementary/Alternative Therapies

Complementary/Alternative Medicine
nccam.nih.gov
www.arthritistoday.org/about-arthritis/types-of-arthritis/
juvenile-arthritis/treatment-plan/natural-and-complementary-
therapies/complementary-therapy-for-juvenile-arthritis

For Pediatric Pain
www.pedspain.ucla.edu/pedpainclinic_therapy
UCLA Laughter Study
www2.healthcare.ucla.edu/pedspain/rp11_rxlaughter.htm
www.rxlaughter.org
Writing as Therapy
www.seedison.com/professional-services-of-suzanne-
edison-psychotherapist-poet-educator/

Education

For specific information on your state's laws, visit the Department
of Education website for your state.
Information on 504 and IEP plans from the Federal Government
www2.ed.gov/about/offices/list/ocr/504faq.html
www2.ed.gov/policy/speced/guid/idea/iep-qa-2010.pdf
Suggestions for 504 Plans
www.arthritistoday.org/about-arthritis/types-of-arthritis/
juvenile-arthritis/daily-life/educational-rights-and-
resources/504-accomodations
www.webmd.com/rheumatoid-arthritis/features/juvenile-
arthritis-at-school-504-plans-ieps-and-pain-issues

General Resources

Questions and Answers about Juvenile Arthritis, NIH Publication
07-4942 (This free booklet contains general information about
juvenile arthritis. It describes what juvenile arthritis is and how
it may develop. It also explains how juvenile arthritis is
diagnosed and treated.)
Catalog.niams.nih.gov
American Autoimmune Related Disease Association
www.aarda.org
American College of Rheumatology
www.rheumatology.org
Arthritis Foundation
www.arthritis.org

www.arthritistoday.org/tools-and-resources for a glossary

Arthritis Foundation/Kids Get Arthritis Too (age-specific tips for kids)

www.arthritistoday.org/kgat/

Childhood Arthritis and Rheumatology Research Alliance

www.carragroup.org

Cure JM

www.curejm.org

Juvenile Arthritis Association

www.juvenilearthritis.org

The International Autoimmune Arthritis Movement

www.iaamovement.org

National Institute of Arthritis and Musculoskeletal and Skin

www.niams.nih.gov

Stop CAID Now!

www.stopcaidnow.org

Medications

To research your child's medications, visit the manufacturers' websites. Many offer welcome gifts, product information, answers to FAQ, nursing support/hotline, or financial assistance programs.

Calendar Blister packaging for travel or convenience (offered through some pharmacies such as Walmart and selected CVS or RiteAid)

www.geriatriccaremanagement.com/2011/01/help-mom-manage-her-medications/

Do-it-yourself blister packaging

www.mts-mt.com/consumers/

Why blister/calendar packaging is a good idea

www.ncbi.nlm.nih.gov/pubmed/10560719

Online Communities

But You Don't Look Sick—Living with a Chronic Illness

www.butyoudontlooksick.com

Creaky Joints (online community and information for people of
all ages with arthritis)
    www.creakyjoints.org
Facebook (search for specific groups)
    www.facebook.com
Wego Health
    www.wegohealth.com/about/about_us

Patient Assistance Programs
    www.needy.meds.org

Products
Buzzy (for pain relief, shots, labs, blood draws)
    www.buzzy4shots.com
MedicAlert (medical ID jewelry)
    www.medicalert.org
My Body Check Journal (for kids/parents to keep track of
JA symptoms)
    bodycheckjournal.com
My RA application for iPhone
    www.trackmyra.com
Pillid (portable pill carrier for water bottles)
    www.thepillid.com
Port-accessible clothing for hospital visits (these are sized for
adults/teens)
    www.ronwear.com
    www.libreclothing.com/clothing.html
SPF Clothing (since sun sensitivity is a problem with some
diagnoses such as JM and certain medications)
    www.coolibar.com
    www.spfstore.com/Kids-sun-protection-swimwear-s/49.htm
Wash-in SPF for clothing (turn your own clothing into SPF wear)
    sunguardsunprotection.com

Research
Center for Disease Control
www.cdc.gov/arthritis/basics/childhood.htm
Google Scholar
scholar.google.com
Johns Hopkins
www.hopkinsmedicine.org
Laboratory Tests Explained
labtestsonline.org
Mayo Clinic
www.mayoclinic.com
MedLine/PubMed Resources
www.nlm.nih.gov/bsd/pmresources.html
National Institutes of Health (NIH)
www.nih.gov
PubMed, PubMed Central, PubMed Health
www.ncbi.nlm.nih.gov/pubmed
www.ncbi.nlm.nih.gov/pmc/
www.ncbi.nlm.nih.gov/pubmedhealth/
Europe PubMed
europepmc.org
PubMed Central Canada
pubmedcentralcanada.ca/pmcc/
(Another great resource is the website for your local children's hospital.)

Other
Stages of Death—Elizabeth Kübler Ross
www.ekrfoundation.org

Appendix

School Letter for Rheumatologic Diseases

Date_____
Student's Name_____ DOB_____
Name of School_____Grade_____
Condition followed for_____

This chronic disease is characterized by joint swelling, pain, stiffness, and fatigue. In addition, this student has
_____.

We recommend the following services be provided by the school:

- ☐ Modified physical education to include:
  - ○ Activities as tolerated
  - ○ No contact sports
  - ○ No repeated stress or pounding of joints
  - ○ No weight bearing on arms or wrists
- ☐ Adaptive physical education
- ☐ No physical education
- ☐ No sitting on floor
- ☐ Rest period in middle of day for fatigue (as needed)
- ☐ No sun exposure between the hours of _____ a.m. to _____ p.m.
- ☐ Two sets of books including workbooks (one for in class and one for home use)
- ☐ Use of elevators (if applicable)
- ☐ Extra time between classes
- ☐ Provision for locker on each floor (if applicable)
- ☐ Modified assignments to include use of tape recorder
- ☐ Computer for taking notes and homework assignments
- ☐ Extended time for assignments
- ☐ No timed tests, including standardized testing
- ☐ Allow to get up and stretch as needed to minimize stiffness
- ☐ Allow use of "fat" pens, pencils & crayons
- ☐ Use of oral tests
- ☐ No grades for handwriting
- ☐ Plan class schedule to minimize amount of walking; cluster classes in close proximity
- ☐ Plan schedule with least demanding class in morning
- ☐ Physical and occupational therapy evaluation to plan accessibility and adaptation needs in school environment (as needed and on a quarterly basis). Please evaluate early in the morning.
- ☐ Dual enrollment: homebound/regular classroom. We request that homebound be implemented if more than three consecutive school days are missed.
- ☐ Individual education plan (IEP) evaluation and implementation
- ☐ 504 plan and staffing
- ☐ Handicapped bus for transportation to and from school
- ☐ May occasionally miss school due to medical appointments or may be absent on days when he/she is having a disease flare. Should not be penalized for these absences and should be permitted to make up all school work missed.
- ☐ Develop an evacuation plan to ensure safe departure from the building, including a location for the student to sit down in shade while waiting outside
- ☐ Please allow bathroom use as often as needed
- ☐ Other:_____
- ☐ Other:_____

Please call if you have any other questions or concerns. Thank you for your assistance and cooperation regarding this student.

Sincerely,

_____
Physician signature

Doctor name:
Address:
Ph #:
Fax#:

Visit www.sprypub.com to download a printable pdf.

Acknowledgments

Writing *Living with Juvenile Arthritis: A Parent's Guide* has been a labor of love. I am not a writer by profession, and five years ago I never imagined I would be an "expert" in this field. The last few years have been a very long and difficult journey for my family, and so many times I wished I had some type of instruction manual to help get me through the next bump in the road.

In 2012, my friend Mia Patterson Brennan approached me with the idea of doing just that for other families in my situation. She introduced me to Lynne Johnson and the staff at Spry Publishing who decided to take a chance on me. With the help of Robin Porter, who collaborated with me every step of the way, I set out to create a comprehensive guide to parenting a child with any of the diagnoses that fall under the JA umbrella. Along the way, I was overwhelmed by the support I received from my friends and family, as well as the families of so many other juvenile arthritis sufferers. But, the support didn't end there: Folks from the medical community, educational arena, and insurance and nonprofit worlds also lent their expertise, helping me to provide accurate information across all areas that a JA family may encounter. To all those who have been so generous with their time, experiences, and stories, I am greatly appreciative.

On a more personal note, I want to extend my sincere thanks to my husband Fred, who allowed me hours upon hours of time alone so I *could* write, and to my mother Ervil, who encouraged me that I *could* do this each day. I never could have done this without your love and support.

On a long list of people who have touched our lives and provided assistance over the years, there are a few who deserve special mention. First, I would like to thank Grant's doctors, especially his pediatrician Dr. Joshua Levin, who has always gone above and beyond the call of duty. I am also grateful for my dear friend Anke Smith, my first hospital "roomie," who introduced me to my first online forum and helped save me from isolation. She took me under her wing at a time when I was feeling lost and has since been an invaluable source of support. Similarly, Monica Forss took an interest in our case and within a short time was helping me with *everything*! As a nurse she's been a valuable resource, but as a friend she has provided middle-of-the-night medical advice and made 50-mile house calls. Both of these women have been central to my JA journey.

Finally, I want to thank my children, Grant and Evan, for selflessly sharing their story with the world. They were patient with *me* while I learned to become a JA mom and, without their support, this book would never exist! Although I never would have chosen this path for them, I am proud of the young adults it has made them become.

Index

501c3 (nonprofit) organizations, 242, 244

——————— A ———————

AARDA. *See* American Autoimmune Related Disease Association
Acceptance stage of grief, 41
AD. *See* Autoimmune disease
Advocacy summit, 239
AF. *See* Arthritis Foundation
Alternative therapy
　for JA treatment, 108
　for pain management, 125
American Autoimmune Related Disease Association
　advocacy activities of, 239
　poster on autoimmunity, 14
Amygdala, 226
ANA. *See* Antinuclear antibody
Anger stage of grief, 40
Anti-cyclic citrullinated peptide (anti-CCP) antibodies, 102
Antinuclear antibody, 103
Arthritis. *See also* Juvenile arthritis; Juvenile idiopathic arthritis; Rheumatoid arthritis
　definition of, 24
　prevalence of, 22
Arthritis Advocacy Summit, 239
Arthritis Foundation, 165, 220, 223
　"Arthritis Ambassadors" for, 239
　501c3 (nonprofit) organizations, 242, 244
　family days, 238
　JIA definition of, 25
　JIA statistics, 27
　local family education day sponsored by, 160
　low-cost events for families to connect, 161, 224
Art therapy programs, 224
Autoimmune disease
　in children, 7
　genetic background of, 6
　healthcare costs of, 7
　pathology of, 6
　prevalence of, 6–7

——————— B ———————

Bargaining stage of grief, 41
Biologic agents, 104
Board-certified practicing pediatric rheumatologists, 22
Brain fog, 177
Bucket list of Grant
　ambitious goals, 231–32
　anticipation of future in, 232
　benefits of, 233
　profound effect on parent, 232
　simple goals, 231
Burnout
　prevention or alleviation of
　　listening child's concern, 196
　　positive thinking, 197
　　reducing the stress load, 196–97
　　spending quality time as family, 197–98
　　stay connected with friends, 197
　warning signs of, 195

——————— C ———————

Canine Compassionate Companions, 244–45
CARRA. *See* Childhood Arthritis and Rheumatology Research Alliance
Catharsis, 226
Cheering section. *See also* JA community, getting involved with
　conferences and camps, 161
　connections for kids, 156–57
　family and friends, 145
　importance in football, 144
　knowing what to say, 146–52
　making connections within JA community, 158–60
　members of, 144
　online community
　　JM Moms and Caregivers, 154–55

shared experiences, 155–56,
  158–60
school as part of, 172–73
strangers
  hospital roommates, 152–54
  kind words, 145–46
Childhood Arthritis and Rheumatology Research Alliance, 248
Childhood, fostering normal. *See also*
  Traveling with JA kids, tips for
  balancing act, 186
  burnout prevention for, 195–97
  caring third party role in, 194–95
  empowerment of JA kids
    fostering independence, 193–94
    inclusion in decision-making
      process, 193–93
  maintaining an element of fun,
    187–89
  making it normal, 185–86
  school for child, 186
  spiritual care, 195
Communication with doctors
  brief, 75
  challenges linked with, 68–69
  educating yourself for, 46
  importance of effective, 72, 83
Complementary therapy, 108
  for JA treatment, 108
  for pain management, 125
*Conquering Your Child's Chronic
  Pain*, 126
Corticosteroids, 93, 104, 163
Counseling
  JA treatment plan, 109–10
  for removal of "unhappy" triggers,
    210–11
Counter-indication accidents, 68
C-reactive protein, 103
CRP. *See* C-reactive protein
Cure JM (organization), 240–41

——————— D ———————
Denial stage of grief, 40

Depression stage of grief, 41
Diet and exercise, 215–16
Doctor's visits, tips for making most
  of, 73
DRESS syndrome, 26, 34
Drug-to-drug interactions, 68–69
Drug trials
  advantages of, 246
  for off-label uses, 248
  participation in
    factors to be considered for, 246–47
    program research for, 246
  specialist recommending, 246, 248
  steps of, 247–49

——————— E ———————
Education, 168
Educational setting, plans used in. *See
  also* School education of JA
  children
  homebound schooling, 172
  individualized education plan, 175–
    76, 182
  504 plans, 174–75
Emotional brain center, 226
EOBs. *See* Explanations of benefits
Erythrocyte sedimentation rate, 103
ESR. *See* Erythrocyte sedimentation
  rate
Explanations of benefits, 80–81

——————— F ———————
Families living with JA. *See* JA families
Family matters
  extended family members
    communication with, 140
    educating, 140
    putting little distance between, 140
    unsolicited advice, 139–40
  healthy relationships, 129
  nurturing marriage relationship,
    130–31
  supporting healthy sibling, 132–37,
    141–43

unsolicited advice, 139
ways to stay connected, 131
Flares
definition of, 110
preparing for, 111–14
distraction, 111–12
hospitalization, 111
warning signs, 110

——————— G ———————
Grief, Kübler-Ross stages of, 40–41
Guilt
"administering meds," 212–13
definition of, 211
letting yourself get lost in, 210
"my baby is sick," 213
"remission," 214
"to medicate or not," 212
"who done it," 211–12

——————— H ———————
Healthcare team for JA
effective communication, 72
finding the right fit, 71–72
management of, 68–69
need to change, 67–68
nephrologist, 67
ophthalmologist, 63–67
pediatrician, 67, 70–71
pharmacist, 68–69
rheumatologist, 63, 70–71
High-5-Club, 242, 249–251
Homebound schooling, 172
Homebound tutoring, 181–82
Hospital stay, tips for making easier
ask for available services, 38
food options, 36
headphones and other gadgets, 37
light packing, 35
pillowcase and blanket, 37–38
planning, 38
spare bag at home, 35
writing everything down, 36–37
Humane Society (no-kill shelter), 244

——————— I ———————
IDEA. See Individuals with Disabilities
Education Act
IEP. See Individualized Education Plan
Individualized Education Plan, 175–
76, 182
Individuals with Disabilities Education
Act, 175
Insurance company
importance in securing right
treatment, 76
tips for working with, 77–82
case managers, 81
denial of claim, 78–79
off-label use of medications, 79–80
read your medical policy, 77–78
review of EOBs, 80–81
up-front information, 79
Internet
blogging, 220–22
information search on, 219–20
Iritis, 64

——————— J ———————
JA. See Juvenile arthritis
JAA. See Juvenile Arthritis Association
JA children. See also JA families
Cameron's journey with JA, 56–58
Connor's journey with JDM, 47–50
diagnosis, 48–49
hospital stay, 49
muscle biopsy, 48
pain in legs, 48
Emily's JA diagnosis, 223
Emi's journey with SOJIA, 95–99
anemic, 96
bi-weekly infusions, 99
episodic fever, 96
ileus treatment, 98
IV cyclosporine, 97
on NSAID, 95
pale and lethargic, 95
pulse steroids administration, 97–98
reaction to steroids, 97

Evan, The Other Kid, 141–43
Evan's JA diagnosis, 27–28, 137–38
    getting involved with JA
        community, 243–44
    JIA symptoms, 28–29
    participation in drug trials, 246
fostering normal childhood of. See
    Childhood, fostering normal
Grant
    considering threshold for activity
        of, 235
    "go-with-the-flow" kind of baby, 17
    JIA symptoms, 29
    participation in drug trials, 246
    participation in medical studies, 245
    as shelter volunteer for Irving
        animals, 243–44
    social outings, 235
Grant, fostering normal childhood of
    avoiding invasive tests for, 196–97
    empowerment, 192–94
    excursions, 187–89
    spending quality time as family,
        197–98
    stay-away camps, 193–94
    stress load reduction, 197
Grant, frustration caused by JA to
    difficulty in playing sports, 202
    doctors, 199
    family members, 201
    medicines, 199–200
    people, 200
    stopped height growth, 202
    weight gain, 201–2
Grant, life lessons by, 198–206
    communication with doctors, 203
    educating people, 203
    empathy, 204
    frustration, 199–202
    hard work for sports, 204–5
    height and weight problems, 203–4
Grant school education, 169
    easing the transition, 176–77
    educational plan, 172–73

teachers and administrators on,
    170–71
Grant's illness
    autoimmune conditions, 45–46
    discomfort and flares, 110–12
    managing family life during. See
        Family matters
    pain levels from JIA, 115–18,
        122–26. See also Pain
        management
    paradigm shift in family with, 42–43
    private blogging about, 221–22
    reaction to rheumatology
        medication, 31–33
    shift in attitude with, 17–18
    steps to cut costs of, 83
    strange gait and discomfort of,
        18–19
    terrible-twos behavior of, 18, 28
    upheaval experienced from, 39–40
Grant's illness and health of parents
    diet and exercise, 215–16
    regular checkups, 215
    stress management, 216–18
Grant's JA diagnosis, 137–38
    allergic reaction, 26, 34
    ankle pain, 20–21, 26
    back pain, 22–23
    communication with doctors, 46
    confirmation of JA, 23–24
    connections with kids, 156–57
    consultation with pediatric
        rheumatologist, 21
    enthesitis-related JIA, 45
    flexible scheduling during, 41–42
    human interaction with kids, 42
    information and support for, 25–26
    readmitted to hospital, 34
    shift in attitude, 17–18
    spondyloarthropathy and, 45
    at Vanderbilt Children's Hospital,
        19–20
    visit to ER doctor, 23, 33–34
guilt with Emma's JA

"administering meds," 212–13
"my baby is sick," 213
"remission," 214
"to medicate or not," 212
"who done it," 211–12
Jenna, A Perfect Fit for, 64–67
Kylie's journey with JIA
    biologics, 164
    blood work, 162–63
    corticosteroid injections, 163
    JA community support, 165–66
    methotrexate injections, 163–64
    pain and inflammation, 162–63
Noah's journey with JA, 58–60
    emotional roller coaster, 158
    online support, 158–60
    social connections, 160
Noah's journey with juvenile
    enthesitis-related arthritis
    blood work and MRI, 51
    methotrexate injections, 52
    mild and intermittent symptoms, 50
    remission status, 53
    steroid injections, 52–53
    swollen lymph nodes, 52
parents roles in Grant's treatment, 10
    considering all sources, 99–101
    questioning doctors, 92–94
    sharing responsibilities, 89–90
    trusting yourself, 90–91
school education of. See School
    education of JA children
staying at home, 169
traveling with. See Traveling with JA
    kids, tips for
Zoe's journey with JA, 53–56
    diagnostic tests, 54–55
    symptoms, 54
    treatment and pain management,
    55–56
JA community, getting involved with
    advantages of, 158–60, 248
    advocacy summit, 239
    AF family days, 238

camps, 237
drug trials. See Drug trials
getting kids involved, 238
    participation in family fun days, 243
    providing "cozies," 243
    shelter volunteers, 243–44
medical studies. See Medical studies
mixing business and pleasure, 239–40
organizations, 237
other families, 238
parents on a mission
    Cure JM, 240–41
    High-5-Club, 242, 249–51
    Juvenile Arthritis Association, 240
    Stop CAID Now!, 240–41
product development, 242
Sharing This Journey, 158–60
Sticking Together, 223–24
volunteer opportunities, 239–40
JA families, 145, 214. See also Family
    matters; JA children
Allie's medical mystery, 61–62
benefits of knowing other, 223–24,
    238
dealing with unsolicited advice, 139
lifelong relationships with, 223–24
list of what to say and what not to
    say for, 146–51
Janis, Byron, 165–66
JA treatment plan
    administering shots at home, 105–7
    cheering section and. See Cheering
        section
    complementary and alternative
        therapies, 108
    counseling, 109–10
    developing own strategies, 29–30
    family matters and. See Family
        matters
    handling of flares, 110–14
    medications for. See Medications for
        JA
    occupational therapy for, 107–8
    physical therapy for, 107

planning, 46–47
routine care, 108–9
steps to cut costs, 83–84
subtypes response to, 45
team approach. *See* Team approach
for JA treatment
JDM. *See* Juvenile dermatomyositis
JIA. *See* Juvenile idiopathic arthritis
JM Moms and Caregivers (Facebook
group), 154–56
JRA. *See* Juvenile rheumatoid arthritis
Juvenile arthritis, 128. *See also* JA
children
common symptoms of, 15, 16
definition of, 44
diagnosis of
calculating the odds for, 26–27
genetic testing, 16
laboratory tests, 15–16, 102–3
support and help for, 9–10
families with. *See* JA families
managing life with. *See* Life with JA,
managing
medications for. *See* Medications
for JA
misunderstanding about, 24
most common form of, 44
pathology of, 6
prevalence of, 27, 44
siblings developing
ages and subtypes of, 29
risk of, 27
systemic or localized, 24–25
treatment plan. *See* JA treatment plan
types of, 25
as umbrella term, 24–25
Juvenile Arthritis Association, 240
Juvenile dermatomyositis, 45
diagnosis of, 48–49
genetic links regarding, 49
Juvenile idiopathic arthritis, 31, 44
categories of, 25
definition of, 25
Juvenile rheumatoid arthritis. *See*

Juvenile idiopathic arthritis

—————————— L ——————————
Life with JA, managing, 128
cheering section. *See* Cheering
section
family matters. *See* Family matters
Lupus, 46

—————————— M ——————————
Macrophage activation syndrome, 97
MAS. *See* Macrophage activation syndrome
Medical checkups of parents, 215
Medical studies, 245–46
Medication dollars, maximizing your,
84
Medications for JA
DMARDs, 104
NSAIDs, 103
side effects of
brain fog, 177
change in appearance, 176–77
weight gain, 176
special care of, during travelling,
190–92
Mental health, 109
Methotrexate injections, 42, 52, 57,
66, 74, 104, 155, 163–64
Mood lifters identification, 208
breaks, 209–10
support systems, 209

—————————— N ——————————
National Arthritis Foundation, 239
Nonsteroidal anti-inflammatory drugs,
20, 29, 56, 95, 97, 103
NSAIDs. *See* Nonsteroidal anti-inflam-
matory drugs

—————————— O ——————————
Occupational therapy, 107
Organizations
Arthritis Foundation. *See* Arthritis

Foundation
Cure JM, 240–41
High-5-Club, 242, 249–51
Juvenile Arthritis Association, 240
Stop CAID Now!, 240–41
OT. *See* Occupational therapy

——————— P ———————

Pain from JA, 115–18
ankle and back, 20–23, 26
difficulty in dealing with, 115–18
emotional and physical effect of, 118–19
and inflammation, 162–63
management of. *See* Pain management
pain in legs, 48
referred to PMC for treatment, 122–26
Pain management, 55–56, 115
cold pack, 116–17
contacting pediatrician, 119–20
pain clinic for. *See* Pain management clinic
rheumatologist and counselor for, 121
Pain management clinic
complementary and alternative therapies, 123, 125
selection of, 122, 126
UCLA program, 122
Grant's pain treatment, 123–26
Parents of children with ADs. *See also* JA families
blogging about children's conditions, 221–22
challenges faced by
adjustments to day-to-day life, 10
dealing with pain. *See* Pain management
frustrations and, 7, 198
as medical caregiver, 10
day-to-day life of
child's threshold for activity, 234–35
control issues in, 228
going with flow of changes, 228–30

right balance, 236
unpredictable and uncertain, 228, 229
variable activities, 229
discovering positive side to JA
adjustments, 233
appreciation of victories, 230
dealing with hard time, 233–34
flexibility with plans, 230
effective communication with doctors, 72
family matters. *See* Family matters
grieving of hope, 208
knowledge of child's condition
information search for, 219–20
stress levels linked to lack of, 218
mood lifters identification by, 208
breaks, 209–10
support systems, 209
physical health of
diet and exercise, 215–16
mood and "feeling" of home environment, 207
paying attention to, 207
regular checkups, 215
stress management, 216–18
removal of "unhappy" triggers by, 209
counseling for, 210–11
guilt and worry, 210–14
roles of, in treatment, 10, 207
considering all sources, 99–101
questioning doctors, 92–94
sharing responsibilities, 89–90
trusting yourself, 90–91
Patient registry, participating in, 248
Pediatric autoimmune conditions, educating yourself about, 46
Pediatrician's wish list, 85–87
Pediatric rheumatologists, 16, 21, 60, 64, 66, 70
board-certified, 22
shortage of, 70–71
Physical health of parents

diet and exercise, 215–16
mood and "feeling" of home
   environment, 207
paying attention to, 207
regular checkups, 215
stress management, 216–18
Physical therapy, 107
Pillid, 242
504 plan (educational plan)
   content and scope of, 174, 182
   directives created for, 175
   purpose of, 175
PMC. *See* Pain management clinic
PT. *See* Physical therapy

——————— R ———————

RA. *See* Rheumatoid arthritis
Rehabilitation Act of 1973, 174
RF. *See* Rheumatoid factor
Rheumatoid arthritis, 44
Rheumatoid factor, 102–3
Rheumatology medication
   reactions to, 26, 32
   side effect of, 177

——————— S ———————

School-based support options, 181–82
School education of JA children
   devising educational plan for, 171–73
   parent, educator, physician role in,
     168, 170–71
   realistic expectations from, 179
   regular attendance benefits, 168–69
   right balance for, 169
   strategies to help facilitate, 180–84
     child's current condition, 181
     coaching for skills, 183–84
     commitment to academics, 182–83
     meeting with building principal,
       180–81
     school-based support options,
       181–82
     social experiences, 183
   working with child's school for

benefits of, 173
easing transition back to school,
   176–79
individualized education plan,
   175–76
open line of communication, 173–
   74
504 plans, 174–75
School letter for rheumatologic dis-
   eases, 259
School strategies, 180–84
Section 504 plan. *See* 504 plan
   (educational plan)
"Shot night," tips for, 105–7
Siblings Discordant for Rheumatic
   Disorders, 245–46
SOJIA. *See* Systemic onset juvenile
   idiopathic arthritis
Spondyloarthropathy, 45
Still's disease, 95
Stockholm syndrome, 152–53
Stop CAID Now!, 240–41
Stress management, 216–18
   finding ways for, 224
   writing for. *See* Writing
Study of Families with Twins, 245–46
Systemic onset juvenile idiopathic
   arthritis, 95–96, 98

——————— T ———————

Team approach for JA treatment
   controlling your emotion, 75–76
   healthcare team. *See* Healthcare
     team for JA
   insurance company. *See* Insurance
     company
   photographic evidence, 74–75
   recording of information, 72–74
"The Spoon Theory," 234–35
Traveling with JA kids, tips for
   care with medications, 190–92
   frequent rest stops, 189
   keeping snacks, 192
   medical supplies, 190

openness to changing plans, 190
schedule modification, 189
time for rest and recovery, 190
Tumor necrosis factor (TNF) inhibitors, 104

———————— U ————————

"Unhappy" triggers, removal of, 209
counseling for, 210–11
guilt and worry, 210–14
Uveitis, 64

———————— W ————————

Writing
and catharsis, 226
experiences of parenting JA child, 225, 227
as form of therapy, 224
medical journal, 222
personal journaling, 222
prefrontal cortex engagement in, 226
releasing feelings with, 226–27
as righting journey, 225–27
therapeutic function of, 225–26

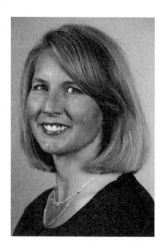

Kimberly Poston Miller is the mother of two children who live with juvenile idiopathic arthritis. Through the management of her sons' chronic illnesses, she has become not only an active and inspired advocate for arthritis awareness, but also a seasoned expert on finding and maintaining balance within a family that is beset by extreme circumstances and often overwhelming challenges.

Robin Porter—With a background in corporate communications, Robin Porter is a versatile freelance writer, who has written a wide variety of materials. Most notably, she has authored several company history/ anniversary books, as well as co-authored books on various medical issues. Robin lives with her husband, Alan, and son, Sean, in Canton, Michigan.

Photo by Don Shepherd, *Tampa, Florida*